PARHAM DONYAI

THE 10 MINUTE MINUTE

BACK PAIN CURE

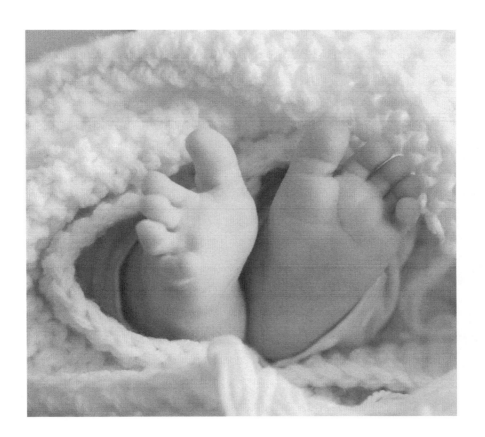

"The feet hold the secret to your health"

The 10 Minute Back Pain Cure

Author: Parham Donyai LLB(Hons), Dip. Legal Practice, MCSR, ITEC
Cover Design: Vilius Musinskas
Copyright (c) 2015
Published by: Active Press
Contact: info@active.gi

DISCLAIMER:

This book is not intended to diagnose, prevent or cure disease. If you have a medical condition, you should seek the opinions of a doctor.

If you get any side effects from any of the advice in this book, you must stop immediately and seek the advice of a doctor.

Nothing in this book is intended to replace the advice and assistance given by a doctor or medical practitioner.

Complimentary medicine is considered a supplement to traditional medical treatment and not a substitute.

Parham Donyai is not a medical doctor and does not claim to be.

If you are going to follow the methods in this book, you are advised to follow as closely as possible and as accurately as possible.

Contents

Preface

I was in Marbella, Spain the other week, talking to a very wealthy friend of my lawyer. He had heard about my Zonal Probing Technique and was very eager to have a few minutes with me.

This man pays £200,000 a year to moor his yacht in Puerto Banus Harbour and never uses it! So you can imagine that he has money and can afford the best medical treatments. He has chronic sinusitis and in fact, has been to some of the best doctors in Spain, Germany, USA and the UK. No doctor has given him a fix or alleviated the problem. He has to permanently carry a corticosteroid bottle and spray it into his nostrils, which is working less and less and he is having to use more and more of it.

I asked him if he had ever tried any dietary changes or any zonal techniques on his feet. He said no. I could see the type of person he was, much like most of us. Comfortable in his "ways". I asked him if he REALLY wanted his sinusitis to go away and whether he was willing to do anything. He said he was desperate.

Over lunch, I could see him starting to sniff and blow his nose as soon as he started on the bread. I told him he needs to come off all wheat and all dairy foods for just 2 weeks to see very positive results. Having worked with many clients with similar problems, I was confident that he would see a dramatic improvement in his sinusitis. He said absolutely no problem and although it will be hard, he will give it a go.

I then asked him if he slept on goose & down feather pillows or synthetic. He said goose feather (which is rare these days!) - a leading cause of sinus/nasal problems for many. I said this needs to be replaced with synthetic. He was not willing to do this. Not even for 2 weeks. It was an absolute no for him!!!

What's my point, you ask? And what does this story have to do with back pain? I will explain...

My point is that you cannot have it all. Before you read this book and start the process to alleviate your back pain, you need to sit down with yourself and make a decision that you are serious about getting rid of your back pain and enough is enough. You need to decide that this is the one time you really will follow it through and that you will not give up on the techniques in this book and you will focus and persevere with everything you will be reading in the following pages. After all, after the initial very reasonable price (in my opinion!) of the book, the rest is free! You won't be paying a therapist a weekly amount and you won't be paying for expensive specialist treatments. You will just be devoting some of your time.

If you can make this promise to yourself and set your mind for it, you will be so glad you did and you will succeed in alleviating your back pain. However you will need to make sacrifices in the form of time, some discomfort and going without certain little daily things that you have been used to. This is the bad news.

The good news is that if you can commit and follow through to the end, in just a few sessions, your back pain will be a thing of the past. So forget about your goose feathers and alike and things that are really not that important in the light of good health and decide that you are going to go for it and give it 100%.

Only then will you be truly successful.

1
About the author
& this book

Parham Donyai LLB (Hons), Dip. Legal Practice, MCSR, ITEC is a qualified Reflexologist and qualified Reflex Zone Therapist. He is also a successful entrepreneur, founder of LA Muscle Sports Nutrition and founder of The Active Channel, Europe's no.1 health & fitness television channel. He is the author of 3 books on the body and hundreds of his articles on Zone Therapy, Reflexology, health & fitness, exercise, diet, nutrition and complimentary medicine have been published around the world since 1993.

Parham Donyai was introduced to and trained in Zone Therapy by the world's leading Zone Therapist, the late Joseph Corvo, the therapist to celebrities and royalty such as Britain's Princess Diana and The Duchess of York. He went on to qualify as a Reflexologist and Reflex Zone Therapist at the Crane School of Reflexology in the early 1990s at a time when mainstream Reflexology was almost unheard of.

Over the years, Parham has been working to perfect and enhance what he has learnt. Parham's proprietary "Zonal Probing Technique" produces amazing results far more rapidly than traditional Reflexology or Zone Therapy. In the 10 Minute Back Pain Cure, Parham shows you his unique technique using specific "Rapid Relief Zones" on the feet for treating most back problems. Parham uses his extensive exercise, diet and nutrition expertise as additional tools to further alleviate your back pain.

Zone Therapy and holistic medicine see back pain very differently from traditional medicine. Doctors like to pin-point where back pain comes from and often classify it with phrases such as a "slipped disc". Zone Therapy sees the back and spinal areas as a whole. If there is a problem with the back, there will be tenderness on the relevant reflex zones of the feet.

The Zonal Probing Technique applies direct pressure in a unique way to very specific Rapid Relief Reflex Zones of your feet which directly communicate with your problematic back areas. Using Parham's technique, you can alleviate your back pain in just 10 minutes. This can be a one-off 10 minutes if it is an acute problem or several 10 minute sessions for chronic back pain. When the tenderness on the relevant points of the feet are worked out, your back pain miraculously disappears.

Whether you have had back pain for years, needed surgery, have had surgery and the pain has returned or have just done something to cause back pain, Parham's Zonal Probing Technique will work for 99% of you. If you persist, you can be totally free of back pain in just a few short weeks. The beauty of this unique Zone Therapy method is that it is very quick-acting, permanent, can be performed in the comfort of your home and best of all it is free.

Parham's Zonal Probing Technique is not practised by anyone else in the world and produces astonishing positive results quite literally "in front of your eyes". Its pin-point accuracy and method of application make it totally unique.

By purchasing this book, you have shown that you are serious and determined to be rid of back pain. Now you need to be persistent and patient and apply the method described here. Your back pain will soon be a thing of the past.

2
What is back pain and the scopes of this book

You are reading this book because you, a loved one or someone you know suffers from back pain. Other than that, perhaps you are curious as to the claim this book makes and want to know more. In either case, I think you will find this book an interesting read and if I have done my job well, you will find it extremely helpful in alleviating back pain for you or others.

The first thing to overcome is obviously your skepticism and if you are like the rest of the population, you will be very skeptical of what I am promising you. Don't worry, I too am very skeptical and logical by nature and it's not easy to convince me of things. But I have been convinced! I was convinced in 1991 and have seen the incredible results Zone Therapy gives for back pain ever since. It really is miraculous, especially so for people that have tried other methods with little or no success. As if Zone Therapy was not miraculous enough, my unique Zonal Probing Technique is even more astonishing in results.

A question that I have been asked is why have I written this book now? There are two reasons for this:

Firstly, I have been perfecting my technique over the years and feel that now, it is at a point where I can truly share a whole array of skills and extra exercise, nutrition and postural rules that will heal your back rapidly. I have perfected the 10 Minute Back Pain Cure using Zonal Probing; a unique method that will produce noticeable results for you in ten minutes.

Secondly, I have had a very busy life up to this point. I was studying law and Zone Therapy in my early twenties, then I worked for a while for others, then I started my sports nutrition company LA Muscle, subsequently I started my television and media companies alongside writing 3 books, producing hundreds of documentaries and health & fitness shows, many property deals and starting a family with the person I love.

A book such as this needs undivided attention by the author. More importantly, I feel, it should only be written when the author feels that they are at the height of their knowledge and what they can share will truly benefit the audience; and by benefit, I mean a "noticeable" benefit.

Also there doesn't seem to be anyone practising Zone Therapy in the manner which I do and there seem to be no technical books on the power of Zone Therapy for healing back pain. People around me and those I have treated over the years have persistently asked me to write a book on what I know about alleviating back pain. No one else knows my Zonal Probing Technique and where the Rapid Relief Reflex Zones are; you are about to find out.

What is back pain?

The majority of back pain is really "lower" back pain, divided into acute, chronic and sub-chronic. There are lots of reasons why someone would have back pain: injury, age, occupational posture, obesity, muscle weakness, heavy lifting and even depressive moods.

Back pain, especially lower back pain is the leading cause of an inactive life, limited activity and absence from work throughout the world. In the UK, lower back pain is the number 1 cause of disability amongst the young contributing to 100 million lost work days per year [1].

In the USA, in 1999, 149 million work days were lost due to low back pain. Up to 26% of US residents are affected by lower back pain and 13.8% by neck pain [2].

In developed countries, the occurrence of low back pain is thought to be between 60-70%. The prevalence for children is lower but it is on the rise,

[1] Croft P et al. The prevalence and characteristics of chronic widespread pain in the general population. Journal of Rheumatology, 1993, 20:710-3.
Guo HR, Tanaka S, Halperin WE, Cameron LL. Back pain prevalence in US industry and estimates of lost workdays. Am J Public Health, 1999, 89(7):1029-1035.

[2] Back Pain Prevalence and Visit Rates: Estimates from U.S. National Surveys, 2002 Spine, 2006 Nov. 1;31(23):2724-7 RA Deyo, SK Mirza, BI Martin

probably due to their lack of outdoor activity, sitting on chairs playing computer games and rising obesity [3].

According to Professor Steve Bevan, Director of the Centre for Workforce Effectiveness at the Work Foundation, "sitting" is the main reason why so many people are now affected by lower back pain in comparison to years gone by.

It is estimated that 44 million workers in the European Union have musculoskeletal problems caused by their workspace. The Work Foundation, part of the UK's Lancaster University puts the cost to the European Economy as a result of bone and joint pain at £200 billion per year.

A study by the Lancet in 2012 found that musculoskeletal disease affected 1.7 billion people worldwide. That is 1.7 BILLION people!

Researchers have found that out of 291 conditions studied in the Global Burden of Disease 2010 Study, lower back pain ranked highest in terms of disability than any other condition. Globally almost 1 in 10 people have lower back pain. Prevalence of back pain is highest in Western Europe rising to an incredible 15%.

Lower back pain is treated commonly with anti-inflammatories and pain killers. Physical therapy, rehabilitation, chiropractic manipulation, osteopathy, corticosteroid injections, acupuncture, massage, ice and biofeedback are other alternatives. The last stop on the train to a possible cure is surgery but surgery rarely fixes lower back pain. Surgery has many risks associated with it and most spine surgeons will tell you about the possibility of nerve damage or even paralysis as a result of back surgery [4].

---

[3] Taimela S, Kujala UM, Salminen JJ & Viljanen T. The prevalence of low back pain among children and adolescents: a nationwide, cohort-based questionnaire survey in Finland. Spine,1997, 22: 1132–1136.
Balague F, Troussier B & Salminen JJ. Non-specific low back pain in children and adolescents: risk factors. Eur Spine J, 1999, 8: 429–438.

[4] Phillips FM, Slosar PJ, Youssef JA, Andersson G. Lumbar Spine Fusion for Chronic Low Back Pain due to Degenerative Disc Disease: A Systematic Review. Spine, 2013, (Phila Pa 1976).

There are newer "technologies" on the horizon. 3D imaging, biomaterials and disc re-nutrition or stem cell therapies are all in the pipeline. None really address the root cause of back pain, which lies in your meridians and your body's electromagnetic field - more later.

Can such a huge global problem be addresses in one book?

Neurolinguistic Programming (NLP) says *"As long as you believe it is impossible, you will actually never find out if it is possible or not."*

Add to that *"as long as you are going to be thinking, you may as well think big!"*

This is how I try and live my life and with this sort of belief, you are open to all possibilities and you remove all restrictions.

It always helps when you are learning something new, to learn from someone you respect and someone whose opinions, experience or credentials you value. Or at least someone that doesn't come across as a complete lunatic!

In answer to the above question, I can categorically tell you that a huge global problem such as back pain and especially lower back pain can be addressed in this book and as you will find out, has been.

The materials in this book are new in many ways but at the same time they are thousands of years old. It is just that they have not been presented to you in an easy to understand, easy to apply and concise format. And of course the Zonal Probing Technique applied to Rapid Relief Reflex Zones of your feet is something novel, very effective, if not revolutionary.

This book mixes the ancient and forgotten technique of Zone Therapy with modern methods that see it work in the 21st Century. Back problems nowadays are different with a great many of them brought about as a result of our sedentary lifestyle and often concentrated in specific areas of the feet. You would have certainly not come across my unique Zonal Probing Technique unless you have been a client of mine.

3
How I was introduced
to Zone Therapy

In 1991, I was studying law at the University of Westminster in London, England. I was young, energetic, ambitious, determined…. and cursed with the worst back pain imaginable.

My back pain had started a couple of years earlier. I cannot remember the exact time but it was when I started weight training and lifting heavy weights in the gym. This coincided with a job in the summer washing cars which required a great deal of bending at odd angles. I think the final straw was one evening when I pushed a car that had broken down and the owner was a rather beautiful woman. I was so charitable in those days!

After that, my back was never the same. I had pain almost all the time and it would be so bad that some days I would just want to stay in bed and not move - though staying in bed was not helping either!

I assume you are reading this book because you or someone close to you suffers from some sort of back pain. As a fellow ex back-pain sufferer I can truly tell you that I feel your pain (or rather I did!). I was there and it really is one of the worst pains in the world - if there is any kind of good pain! That constant dull, aching, annoying, crippling pain. If you are lucky, you may get it periodically and then it somehow goes away and if you are unlucky, it is always there. For some, it means you cannot live your life as you deserve.

Back pain comes in many shapes and forms from upper back/neck pain, to lower back pain which can go into the legs in the form of sciatica or compressed nerve. Many people get problems with their legs, hips, nerves and worse, some cannot move or walk or basically, enjoy life.

The route to a so-called cure in the traditional sense is pretty much the same for most people. They visit their doctor and they are offered pain killers, anti-inflammatories, physiotherapy, corticosteroid injection, massage, osteopathy and even surgery. Luck being on your side, one or more of these methods will offer you temporary, semi-permanent or even permanent relief. For many people, back-ache becomes part of their life and they just cannot break the cycle of pain and get back to how they used to be. Even if it goes away for a while, it often comes back. Many people just cope and learn to live with it. That's a shame and I intend to show you that this is not an option if you are truly serious and want to get well.

Hang in there and keep reading. Hope is around the corner and you will find that this book will actually offer you a free, permanent and effective solution.

I went through the whole lot, short of surgery. Even in those days when my knowledge was next to zero, I knew I didn't want to have surgery on my back. I had anti inflammatory pills, I went to see several physiotherapists, I had massage, I had acupuncture, I eventually had a corticosteroid injection in my spine. Nothing worked.

By 1991, I had pretty much gotten used to living a life with constant back pain. I hadn't stopped searching for a cure but with lack of money, needing to study and the Internet not having been born, there was not a huge deal I could have done. I went to University and tried to cope with my back pain as best as I could.

The human body has a remarkable ability to "cope". I don't want you to cope. I want you to get well and that's why I have written this book. You will see that if you follow what I tell you in this book, you will no longer need to cope with a sub-standard, pain-ridden life. You can go on and live your life as it was planned for you and enjoy everything the way you imagined before your back pain.

One of the women in my law class was a very interesting doctor. Her name was Anna Brocklebank and she was about 10 years older than me. One day we were talking about various things and somehow my back pain got into the conversation. In addition to being a doctor, she was very knowledgeable on a great deal of things and seemed to be very well connected to "high society". She was also very eccentric and a real character!

Anna told me to go and see a man named Joseph Corvo.

"He will fix your back", she said.

It's funny but I remember her saying this as if it was yesterday. Now, I know that when she said it, she actually believed that sentence to be true and a promise that was 100% genuine. At the time, I probably thought the same as what most people would think when someone tells them this. I was skeptical and took her promise and certainty with a pinch of salt - a big pinch!

When I met Joseph Corvo, the therapist to celebrities and Royalty

Joseph Corvo (Joe) is probably in the top 2 of the most interesting people I have so far met in my life. He was a Yorkshire man who had been an opera singer and somehow got into Zone Therapy and found that he had a knack for it. I would call it more than a knack. Some people are truly gifted. I would say Joseph Corvo was a healer. I don't mean the hocus-pocus type. He was very knowledgeable, knew how to apply his knowledge accurately, knew human psychology, was charming, had an obvious vast amount of experience in his field and was extremely positive. This amazing positivity comes from the person's inner core as well as the success of that person in their past endeavours - i.e. their experiences. I know about it as I also possess a similar temperament.

When you have done something so many times and been successful at it, you will be very positive and can afford to come across as over-confident. As far as I am concerned (and probably Joe) the client/patient's skepticism is "their" problem, not the therapist's!

I get it. It is a big leap for most people to think that their long term, chronic back pain which no doctor seems to alleviate is going to magically disappear with a few sessions of Zone Therapy on their feet! I was just as skeptical prior to experiencing it for myself; believe me. This is why I am going into some depth in this chapter of when I was "first" introduced to Zone Therapy. I was not born into it. I did not know about it. I did not believe in it. I probably wouldn't have even tried it if someone had explained it to me first! I was skeptical, just like you.

I would like to refer to Joe as a Healer, if that doesn't put you off him. He was more than a therapist. He had a unique gift and in many years since, I have not seen it in any others... well apart from myself, but that's for other people to judge.

Joe used to practice out of his flat in Cleveland Square, London W2. At the time when I first met him, he was treating Princess Diana several times a week, as well as the Duchess of York and actress Rula Lenska to name a few. He was in high demand with politicians, actors and Royalty.

Here is where it gets interesting and you get to see what I mean about this amazing man. He had this huge gift, he was brilliant at what he did, he spent time with you, never rushing you or making you feel like you are on a clock, charmed the hell out of you, got to be your friend and healed your most chronic and persistent problems, fast and wait for it... he only charged £7 per session! Isn't that unbelievable? I mean, this man could have charged hundreds of pounds especially from his rich high profile clients but he charged the same for everyone. A session with the amazing Joseph Corvo would set you back all of seven pounds sterling!

There I was on my first visit, walking up the stairs of this old Victorian building and reaching Joe's door. I knocked and a beautiful lady in her forties answered the door. Her name was Victoria and she had a wonderful French accent. She was Joe's wife. She took me to one of the rooms and sat me on the bed. All was well so far. Lovely flat, charming wife, very relaxing and professional. Then she said: "Take your shoes and socks off. Joseph will be with you shortly!".

I can honestly tell you that in that instant, I really thought I had mis-heard. I continued to sit on the bed and firmly kept my shoes and socks on! What on earth was going on? I was there to try and fix my back and this crazy lady was asking me to take my shoes and socks off. It just didn't make sense.

Joe entered the room a few minutes later. I clearly remember the first time I met Joseph Corvo. He had instant charm and was ultra-friendly. He looked to be in his early sixties, was lean, had solid pec muscles and was clearly hugely more youthful than his actual years; in mind and physical appearance. Of course the first thing he asked was why I "still had my shoes and socks on!".

In 1991, Reflexology was something that most people, including myself had not heard of. Zone Therapy was even more obscure. Zone Therapy was what Joe practiced. The idea of working on your feet to fix a problem in your body was just preposterous in 1991 - and to a large extent still today. When Anna Brocklebank told me to go and see Joe, she sounded so confident that I didn't even bother asking any more questions. I just assumed that he was some super-duper ordinary medical doctor. I would never ever in my wildest dreams imagine that he was someone that wanted to work on my feet to fix my back. How ludicrous was that? As it turned out, it was a turning point in my back pain and my life... as I hope this book will be in your back pain and life.

Joe asked me about the history of my back pain, how it started, what I had done to fix it, how it was during the day, in the mornings, at night and so on. He didn't actually ask me where my back-ache was, which I found strange but now I know why. He didn't need to! He could tell in an instant from my feet!

Joe had this little wooden self-made pointed piece of wood (which I will refer to as a probe from now on) that he used on people's feet to treat their conditions. He started probing my feet with it. He instinctively knew where to press and told me where my backache was within 30 seconds. He was absolutely correct, it was my lower back, more to the right side and would sometimes go down to my leg. As he started pressing harder on the more tender parts of my feet, the pain on my feet started to become unbearable but I have a relatively high pain threshold so I tried hard not to scream out loud! Besides, I was a body builder and had to act tough!

Joe worked on my feet for about 20 minutes. He would put his probe on a spot, rotate it, press harder, go to a different area, come back to the painful tender area, press harder and so on. His main concentration was on the painful areas on the lower side of my right foot and I could see that he was sort of teasing the pain out by keep coming back to it and pressing a little harder every time.

I can honestly tell you that the pain he was giving me was probably worse than my back pain. Actually, he wasn't giving me the pain as such. He was fixing my problem but it was painful. I want to emphasise this point because further down the line you will see that this is not the practitioner giving you pain but more a result of your problem and the practitioner working to alleviate it.

In subsequent sessions with Joe, I sometimes would scream out loud. At times, it was just too much no matter how tough I was - or thought I was! I dread to think what his neighbours thought was going on in his flat but I guess they were probably used to it! I can't imagine that I was the only person that screamed and shouted the place down.

You may ask, why would someone let another person give them so much pain with the "hope" that this may fix their long term back pain? The answer in my mind is a very simple one: because I trusted Joe. From the very first time I met him, I trusted him and this is what I mean when I say he was one of the most interesting, charismatic, knowledgeable and trustworthy individuals I had ever met. For me, there was no doubt that he knew what he was doing and that what he was doing would work for me. The pain was just part of the process and I had to endure it. It's an old adage but no pain, no gain!

I want to emphasise this pain part a little bit to you. Over the years, I have worked on many people and the majority of them have a mid to low pain threshold so when the going gets tough on their feet, they just don't want to have any more treatment or they give up. If there is one thing I have learnt from Joe and Zone Therapy is that the discomfort of the probe working on the tender areas of the feet is a necessary part of the treatment, especially if you want quick and miraculous results. I can easily press lighter and turn the session into a light relaxing massage but that will not fix your back pain in record time and for good. Joe knew this better than anyone. Don't get me wrong, if you really can't take the pain of the probe on your feet, you/your partner/the therapist can press lighter and you will still see results but it will take a little bit longer for your back pain to go - it will still go.

Whether you have a low or high pain threshold, by working on your feet using Zone Therapy and pressing on the tender reflex zones, you will alleviate back pain. The lighter you press the probe, the longer it will take for it to work.

Joe was a patient and understanding man. He would explain over and over again that it is important to push the relevant areas as hard as tolerable. The aim here is not to "give pain to the patient"; far from it. The aim is to balance the body out and remove the blockages that are preventing the body from healing. However, this process does involve pressing hard on the relevant areas of the feet and because these areas are problematic and tender to touch, there will be some pain.

As an example, if someone has a back problem on the left side of their body, they will find that pressing on the back reflex zones of the right foot will not cause them as much discomfort and pain as the left side. It will be the corresponding reflex zones of the left foot which will be tender; left side of the back, left foot. Right side, right foot. This is probably one of the best proofs to those skeptical of Zone Therapy!

I will explain to you in detail a little later on what is Zone Therapy, what is my unique method of Zonal Probing, how it works and why this Method is an amazing evolution from the Joseph Corvo method and how it can produce such amazing results. Joe penned several books on the subject of Zone Therapy and some of them went on to become quite popular. Though informative, the books were more graphic-based and did not really explain a whole amount on why you should try Zone Therapy (if you were skeptical) and none of them covered what I will be covering with you in this book, which includes exercises, diet and postural guidance as additional tools in your journey to back pain obliteration!

How my back pain was fixed for good

During that first session, I could see that as Joe was pressing his probe on my foot, he was having to press just slightly harder after a while to get the same level of pain (and screaming!) out of me. This was interesting to me. His probe was getting rid of the pain on my feet. But how about my back?

I went home that day and thought a lot about what had happened in Cleveland Square. Jo, Victoria, their beautiful apartment, the theory of Zone Therapy that Joe explained to me, how he planned to get rid of my back pain, his unbelievable confidence and of course, the pain he managed to inflict on my feet with that silly little wooden probe of his! What pain!

An unexpected thing happened the day after my first visit to Joe's apartment. My back pain was visibly reduced. It wasn't gone, but I would say it was down by 20-30%. I know it sounds amazing and too good to be true but it was a fact.

My next appointment was a week away so I went back to University and got on with my life that week. My back pain continued to stay at this 20-30% lower level during that week. Needless to say, I was very happy and optimistic. Joe had told me not to do any exercises that week apart from sit-ups in a specific way, which I will describe to you later.

Exercise is great for reducing obesity and for reducing inflammation in your back. Exercise as a whole is anti-inflammatory, which is good for back pain [5].

However whilst you are doing Zone Therapy on your feet to try and reduce inflammation, to open up the meridians and alleviate your back pain, it is a good idea not to exercise. Over-exercising has been shown to increase inflammation in the body [6].

More on inflammation later.

I was heavily into bodybuilding in those days and had a decent set of shoulders and arms. On my next visit to Joe's apartment, he complimented me on my shoulders! I told him I was bodybuilding and that's when I saw a different side to Joe. He was very much into physical culture and had known the great Charles Atlas, one of the early pioneers of mainstream bodybuilding. Joe and I started talking about Charles, Arnold Schwarzenegger, Steve Reeves and all the bodybuilding greats. Joe had known many of them and knew so much about bodybuilding, which was my big passion at the time.

It is fair to say that Joe and I hit it off and liked talking to each other. Later he would show me exercises I could do at home with no weights which would increase the size of my arms, chest and shoulders. He was a great mentor in so many ways and was always so happy and positive. You just don't see people like him very often.

Joe worked on my feet again with his probe and yes, the pain was unbearable again - at times! He would break the session by talking about weight training, keeping fit & strong and would show me more home exercises he recommended for keeping a strong and lean body.

---

[5] Woods JA, Vieira VJ, Keylock KT: Exercise, inflammation, and innate immunity. Neurol Clin 2006; 24(3): 585-99.
Bruunsgaard H: Physical activity and modulation of systemic low-level inflammation. J Leukoc Biol 2005; 78(4): 819-35.

[6] Angeli A, Minetto M, Dovio A, Paccotti P: The overtraining syndrome in athletes: a stress-related disorder. J Endocrinol Invest 2004; 27(6): 603-12.

Joe could see that I was very interested and curious about what he was doing so he started explaining it in more detail. He would tell me how he became interested in Zone Therapy, what his particular technique is and why it worked and would show me why his technique was super-effective. He also said that many people that he worked on did believe him to be a healer because of the way he was able to rid them of their ailments. He never said he himself thought he was a healer. Others did!

I am very sure that Joe did not think much of Reflexology, which he would see as slightly inferior to his Zone Therapy method and his probe. He never said this as such but it was clear that to him, only his Zone Therapy and use of the probe gave incredible results. The pressure and precision of the probe was much more powerful than the weak fingers of Reflexologists, but more later.

This book is about ridding you of back pain. However, Joe worked on and treated many different conditions successfully using the same probe and the same Zone Therapy methods. I have of course worked on and treated many people using Zone Therapy over the years from sinus congestion, to intestinal problems, migraines to more serious conditions but for the purposes of this book, we will stick to back pain.

When I explain my Zonal Probing Technique in more detail later, you will understand what I mean about it being the big daddy to Reflexology. Don't get me wrong, I am qualified in Reflexology and love Reflexology and think it is amazing and very powerful. However, Zone Therapy and in particular, Zonal Probing is far more superior and effective, especially for certain chronic conditions. I would say this method next to Reflexology for back pain for example is like comparing a Ferrari to a Ford. Zonal Probing is the top of the range when it comes to fixing problems within the body through the feet.

The following day after my second session with Joe, I had even less back pain. That horrible, numbing early morning back pain that I used to get upon waking up was now down by around 40-50% and it stayed like that for the rest of the week.

I saw Joe for a number of weeks. In actual fact, my back pain was totally gone after about the 4th session. By this time he was pressing his probe very hard into my foot and the pain and screaming had subsided substantially!

I continued to see Joe because firstly I wanted my back pain to never return again, so didn't consider a few more £7 sessions a big dent in my finances. However, more than anything, I wanted to talk some more to Joe and learn from him. This yearning for knowledge from him was more so, seeing that he and I got on and he was very willing to impart his methods and knowledge to me.

I am not sure whether he conversed and spent so much time with others as I have not been party to all his sessions! All I can tell you is that our bond of bodybuilding and my extreme and obvious interest in exactly what he was doing, enthused Joe to teach me more about what he knew.

This teaching was not in the form of a classroom. He would teach me as he went along working on my feet and would answer all my questions. One of the most important things that eventually came out of our sessions was my own wooden probe...

After a few sessions, I could see that a big part of Joe's method was his wooden probe. One day I decided to chop off the end of a wooden broom handle and try and shape it as close as possible to what Joe was using to treat people. I took my work of art to him and he was very impressed with my efforts and showed me how to perfect the end to get the best results. Joe must have used his own probe on thousands of feet over the years. I too have now had my probe, shaped by the world famous Joseph Corvo for many years and still continue to use it on people who I occasionally treat.

I believe Joe's probe had become an extension of him and I can say the same for my probe too! Using it over so many years, I can feel people's problems through the probe. Please don't read this and think I am giving you some sort of superstitious talk as I am far from superstitious. I am just letting you know that this uniquely shaped wooden probe can let me know of problems as good as if I were to put my fingers on a certain zone of the foot - if not better in some instances, where the fingers cannot get into.

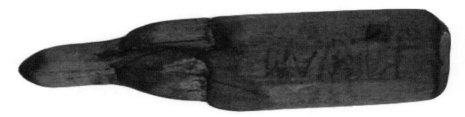

My Zone Therapy Probe, shaped by Joseph Corvo and in use since 1991. It's not pretty but boy is it effective!

I went on to buy all of Joe's books over the years and kept in touch with him occasionally in those early years. One of my life's regrets is that I didn't keep in touch with him more often. This is especially so when I heard that he had passed away peacefully in his sleep in 2012. It would be just like Joe to pass of natural causes and not through any form of major disease. RIP Joseph Corvo, one of the most amazing people that walked this earth.

What I took away from my encounters with Joseph Corvo was not just the "method" he used or the probe he sculpted for me but was something far more powerful and useful; it was the "way" he conducted himself and that amazing confidence and trust he instilled in you. If you meet me in person and especially when I talk about Zone Therapy, you will see what I mean.

When you are young and inexperienced in many things in life, it is not easy to be confident about big subjects such as treating people's chronic problems. However, my life changed following my meetings with Joe and I became extremely confident in Zone Therapy. I was not qualified in it, but I felt more qualified than most professionals (not that there were or are any major Zone Therapists in the world!) because I had learnt from the master and not only had I been shown the methods, I had personally experienced the healing powers of Zone Therapy through the healing hands (and probe) of the best out there. My back pain was gone, I had knowledge that pretty much no one else had and a whole new door had opened for me, leading me to where I am today.

Joseph Corvo cured my back pain. He didn't relieve it, help it or reduce it. He cured it, period. It never came back again. Sometimes I may get a little bit of a problem if I lift heavy or sleep wrong and I know exactly how to fix it in a few minutes. I say this because nothing is fixed forever if you start doing the wrong things. If you don't do any movement or exercise, sleep on a bad bed, develop a huge belly, lift heavy, bend down too fast or do something that's not good for your back, then obviously you may get a back-ache! I cannot guarantee against future negligence, bad luck or accidents!

Zone Therapy only fixes things up to the point of fixing them and ensures that they don't return as long as you stick to some basic principles which will be covered later in this book. These extra helpers which will be explained later will speed up your healing and are the secret added ingredients I will be sharing with you a little later.

My life with a pain-free back

I was grateful to Anna Brocklebank for recommending Joe and of course felt extremely happy that my back pain was gone. Looking back, maybe I should have been even more grateful than I was. I guess I was young and didn't realise that something like that horrible back problem could have become a lifelong debilitating thing, had it gone on. I have met and worked on so many people whose lives have been terribly affected by back pain. I didn't see Anna after our law degree course but always remembered her and her eccentric ways!

Even though I was not qualified as a Zone Therapist, I decided to put some adverts in the local papers and start treating people's back pain using my probe and what I had learnt from Joe. Looking back, it was a brave move.

Here was this young guy (me!), showing up at your house with his wooden probe, no insurance, no formal qualifications in Reflexology or Zone Therapy and he would go on and fix your back pain! I was good at it and started to get recommendations from people.

It was not easy though. Reflexology (or Zone Therapy) was pretty much unheard of and not known in the public psyche. I had a very hard time convincing people of my methods and was always on the back foot (pardon the pun!), especially in those early days. Sometimes it almost felt like I had to pay "them" for the privilege of them letting me fix their problem with my unconventional ways! Everyone was so skeptical and you know what was the worst thing of it all? They would get well, their back pain would subside or disappear but they almost always would say that they weren't sure it was the Zone Therapy. This was very annoying.

People are funny; they forget so easily. Here I was, treating someone that had had a chronic back problem for say 10 years and after a few sessions and them seeing great results, they would say that the problem would have gone away anyway or that they weren't sure it was due to my treatment!

This, I now know is no reflection on my methods or success. It is just the human condition. When we get well, we forget how unwell we were! We are also programmed to have great respect for traditional medicine, doctors and pills but very little appreciation and respect for natural, non invasive methods.

I used to get frustrated by this but then I guess it didn't really matter. I was getting paid relatively good money for those days, £30-£40 for 30 minutes and gaining a great deal of experience. I was very outgoing and totally passionate about my healing powers and Zone Therapy method and knowledge and would pretty much work on anyone and everyone.

My party trick was to get a hold of people's hands and tell them what was wrong with them by just touching their hands. This is because the reflex zones for your body parts and organs are not only on your feet but on the hands too. People loved it - many were freaked out by it! Many would not admit to it if I was doing it in public and it was some problem such as constipation but would later admit to it in private with great amazement. I remember once I told a guy in Nicosia, Cyprus that I could not feel his right kidney (from his hands) and to his (and my) astonishment, he told me that's because he doesn't have a right kidney! I should have had my own TV show!

Over the years, I have worked on many people including several who had had such bad back problems that they had resorted to surgery. None of their back problems had been relieved from surgery permanently, so there I was fixing their backs from their feet in record time. It was unbelievable really. A young guy, with no formal qualifications was doing something that surgeons with many years of training could not do. I am not claiming to be some form of guru by the way. I just learnt the correct Zone Therapy method very well and had a knack for applying it well and beyond that, I was enthusiastic and didn't believe in the word no - a word that I still don't believe in!

I carried on with my legal studies and went on to work as a lawyer for a while. Zone Therapy was never going to be a career for me. It was always on the side-lines and it sure helped make life easier for me on the financial and life experience side. I was being recommended to different people following my early success and soon I didn't have to advertise any more. I was meeting so many interesting people. I can't say that I wanted a life of working on people's feet and hands but I did find the holistic medicine thing very fascinating and would always try and up my knowledge on it.

People who know me, will tell you that I am obsessed with all things to do with the body, Reflexology, Zone Therapy, nutrition, supplements, health, fitness and exercise. I was back then and still am 25 years on…

How I became qualified as a Reflexologist

Although I knew my destiny was not to work on people's feet all my life, I felt that I needed to be formally qualified in what was now a big part of my life. I was going out there, treating serious conditions with no qualifications. It was all getting a little too out of hand!

One time I managed to get a paralysed person's feet moving. It was scary for the relatives, the doctors and even for me! It was time to get qualified.

Joseph Corvo didn't offer any official training and to be honest, I felt I had learnt all I needed to learn from him. I was actually perfecting what he had shown me and getting even quicker results. There was no one teaching Zone Therapy and I really believed no one could teach me more than what I knew already. The only option was to become qualified in Reflexology. I researched many schools and eventually decided to go to the Crane School of Reflexology.

The principal was a most wonderful woman called Beryl Crane. She used to hold her classes with the help of her ever-present fully supportive husband Reg, who I am sad to say has since passed away.

Beryl Crane was extremely knowledgeable and her school was probably the best Reflexology school in the UK at the time. She was the president of the biggest Reflexology Society and would regularly travel and speak in places like China. She went on to pen several Reflexology books including what is probably the definitive manual for Reflexology which is taught in most Reflexology schools.

I liked Beryl a lot. She was very professional, very kind and was a great teacher. I remember, as knowledgeable as she was, even she was very interested in what I had learnt from Joseph Corvo! I didn't mind sharing what I knew of Joe's methods with her. I think I even arranged for her to see Joe once but don't recall what came of it.

I gained some of the highest grades in Reflexology and qualified in Reflexology, Reflex Zone Therapy and anatomy and physiology. To me, these qualifications were icing on a cake that I had already well and truly cooked and was very happy with! It was great to be officially qualified as a Reflexologist but if I was to be honest, I would always revert back to Zone Therapy in practice (and still do). I always had my probe with me! It was just so much more powerful and effective and would give such quick results. I didn't know it at the time but I was developing my own technique.

If I had been smart, I should have done Reflexology on people. It would take longer to produce results, thus giving a better more long term income to me! But I was and have always been too impatient. I want results fast and wanted the same for my clients.

I knew that my own method of Zone Therapy with my wooden probe would produce results way over and above Reflexology, especially with certain ailments such as back and shoulder pain. I was seeing it work amazingly fast on a daily basis.

I continued to practice on people in different countries, in some Expos as a special guest and wrote many articles on the subject. I was never in the mainstream as such because I never saw myself as a full time Reflexologist or Zone Therapist. It was always more a passionate hobby for me rather than a career. However I was in demand!

Having qualified as a Reflexologist and subsequently as a lawyer, I decided that these professions were not for me and that they would never give me the lifestyle I was destined to have! I would practice on people but only when I had time.

I left law in 1997. I was still very passionate about the body, fitness and bodybuilding and started my own company called LA Muscle shortly after, with £5000 savings which I had earned from my Zone Therapy practice.

I don't want to go on too much about my business and entrepreneurial life as it is really not that relevant to this book, however I do need to mention that LA Muscle and my subsequent other ventures such as The Active Channel and many property deals went on to make me a great deal of money. I have been very fortunate and have had great success in business and luckily continue to do so.

My business and financial success is public record so you can check it out for yourself, though I am a private person and tend to be a little bit more low key than I probably should be! Why I am telling you this is because I want you to understand that the reason why I have written this book for you is not financial. I have written this book because it has been something that has been on my mind and I have been meaning to do for many years. The knowledge and exclusive Zonal Probing Method I am going to give you in this book will help you and many others like you who suffer from back pain so it is my responsibility and duty to share it with you. As simple as that.

After my training in various Zone Therapy and Reflexology disciplines, I went on to have quite a successful few years as a Zone Therapist. As an inquisitive and observant person, I started to note down what parts of Zone Therapy work well and what parts need tweaking. I would note down what Reflex Zones were most effective for certain conditions.

Over the years, I started perfecting my own technique which I termed Zonal Probing. I went on to use Zonal Probing on many people and found that by accessing specific points, they would heal and get better faster. I termed these zones "Rapid Relief Reflex Zones" (or Rapid Relief Zones). These were different to those recommended by Reflexologists and Zone Therapists.

The results from Zonal Probing on specific Rapid Relief Zones are incredible. The back and spine have some very precise zones which can be worked on using Zonal Probing for almost miraculous results in as little as 10 minutes. You will be learning these a little later.

4
What is Zone Therapy
and how
does it work?

Zone Therapy is the number one natural non-invasive method for treating 99% of acute and chronic back pain. Top that with the fact that it's free! Can you see why it is not endorsed by doctors, surgeons and not big in the public domain? Something which would make billions of pounds worth of pain killers and pharmaceutical drugs unnecessary!

I am not going to make a big issue or conspiracy theory here but consider the following: If your chronic back pain could be treated by you in your home with no drugs or medical intervention in as little as a few weeks, then where would that leave doctors, surgeons and the pharmaceutical giants that have a big say in many things that go on in the world? What would it do to their profits? And I am asking you this as a capitalist that is partially on the side of the big companies! There is a big interest in not making a big deal out of Zone Therapy and bringing it to the masses or just brushing it off as unscientific hocus pocus with no proof.

How does Zone Therapy work? How does Zonal Probing differ? I will explain Zone Therapy in this chapter and will explain more on Zonal Probing, which is accredited to me in the next chapter. On the one hand I will explain to you exactly how Zone Therapy works shortly. On the other hand, no one knows! As with most complimentary therapies, no one can really pin-point how they work. I know there are theories and many of them make perfect sense but there is also a greater universal "something" out there that governs many things including the healing powers of the body.

Take the brain for example. Scientists know so much about it, yet they know little to nothing about it in some senses. They can tell you that from the perspective of an MRI, this or that part of the brain has a problem. Yet they cannot explain why the same problematic area of the brain can start functioning again through methods such as physiotherapy, repetition or just the passing of time. They can give you theories such as the recent neuroplasticity theory, but they cannot give you certainty.

With the above in mind, I will explain to you how Zone Therapy works and the theories behind it but I am also open-minded enough and have lived enough and seen enough to tell you that no explanation as to the workings of Zone Therapy is comprehensive and definitive.

You could have had the worst MRI of your spine or been told that your vertebrae is gone or your disc is slipped or whatever. Zone Therapy can help you and in many cases heal you. How do you explain that? We can go some way in explaining it and I will do so shortly, but ultimately many things in this world are not black and white or easily explained - especially when it comes to the body.

Zone Therapy dates back to the Egyptians and the Chinese and has been around for thousands of years in some form or other. There is evidence of foot and hand Zone Therapy in China and Egypt dating back to 4000 B.C.

Zone Therapy was "Westernised" by an American doctor called William Fitzgerald who divided the zones of the body into 5 vertical zones on each side of the body, running down and corresponding to the fingers and toes.

Dr Fitzgerald's Zone Therapy was made more mainstream by his assistant, Dr Edwin Bowers. Later in the 1930s and 40s, Dr Eunice Ingham mapped the whole body on the hands and feet; i.e what is now known as Reflexology.

There are many methods, practitioners, maps of the body and lots of confusing literature on Reflexology, Zone Therapy and the differences between the two (if any, according to some). I am going to try and simplify it for you and explain what the difference between Reflexology and Zone Therapy is and how each works and what are the benefits and disadvantages of each. I feel that I am in a good position for doing this as firstly, I was shown real Zone Therapy by one of the best practitioners of it and I have also learnt and been qualified in Reflexology by one of the best practitioners of that too! In addition, I have been practising both since the early 1990s and have perfected my own unique technique of Zonal Probing for speedier recovery.

In a nutshell, your whole body is mapped out on your feet. The toes represent the upper areas such as the head, brain, sinuses etc. The upper part of your feet represent the chest areas, middle part of your feet are the middle region of your body such as your liver and the lower parts are your intestines.

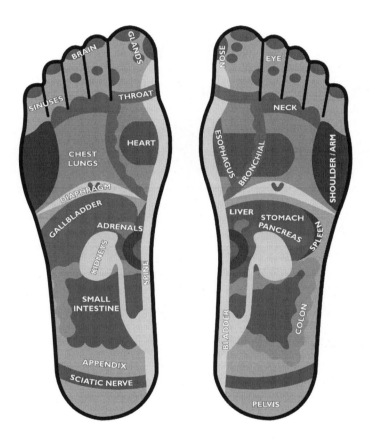

The organs which sit on the right side of your body, will be on your right foot and the organs on the left of your body will be represented on your left foot. If an organ is in the middle or more to one side of your body, this is reflected in the feet too. For example, the liver is on the right, and so represented on the right foot. The spleen is on the left side of the body, so represented on the left foot.

When there is a problem with an organ or area of the body, this is reflected in the corresponding area/s of the feet. It will usually be in the form of tenderness, painful to touch or the feeling of tiny granules under the skin (if you press that area of the foot with your fingers). For example, if you have a cold or a problem with you kidneys, you will find that bang in the centre of both your feet (as you have 2 kidneys) will be painful to touch. The pain will vary according to many things such as severity, duration of the problem, thickness of your skin and your own pain threshold.

There are several theories as to what this pain or feeling of tiny granules under the skin is. The governing theory is that there is a problem in the relevant area of the body. Of this, there is no doubt and every Reflexologist will agree on this one point.

Where it gets a little bit more uncertain is what exactly do the tenderness or the granules represent? Some believe that this is a problem with the electromagnetic field of the body and hence the tenderness on the feet - where it effectively ends up. Others believe the granules are toxins that have gathered around the reflex point of the feet and thus interfering with the body's normal functioning.

In a way, it is neither here nor there whether they are toxins or electromagnetic blockages. I know that Joseph Corvo believed these to be toxins. I do not agree with Joe on this point. I can not see how they can be toxins. I know the theory is that gravity pulls the toxins down and therefore these toxins need to be dispersed with Zone Therapy but I don't think they are toxins. This doesn't explain how very healthy or sometimes very young humans have tenderness and granules on the problematic reflex points. These people are not particularly toxic!

The more plausible theory for me is the electromagnetic field one. I really do believe that the body does have an electromagnetic field of some sorts and I believe it is connected up and down around the body. I like to refer to the end points of this field on your hands and feet as "earthing" and I believe when you get a problem, this affects the earthing of the field and subsequently affects the organs and body parts that are within that affected field.

The fact that the body has its own electromagnetic field is a matter of science. You may have heard of electrocardiogram (ECG) and electroencephalograph (EEG) tests for the heart and brain, respectively.

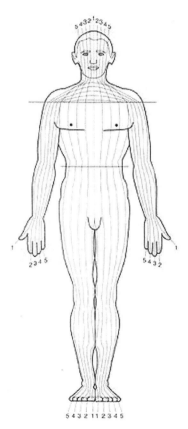

The 5 Meridian lines on each side of the body, running down to the end of the fingers and toes

They measure electromagnetic activity! The fact that there is some sort of electromagnetic field in the body is of no doubt and doctors agree with this. In fact, it can be measured extremely accurately. The electromagnetic activity of the heart is some 60 times the amplitude of brain waves.

When these activities die, we die! When they are impaired, we suffer from disease. When they are restored, we get well. Electromagnetic energy controls the body's chemistry. If our electromagnetic energy is disrupted, our cell metabolism begins to get impaired function.

The body's electromagnetic field protects against disease by improving circulation and repairing the body on a cellular level.

When you work on the reflex points of the feet which are tender or contain granules and you disperse them or work the tenderness out, the body somehow seems to start functioning better again and heals itself. The below par electromagnetic field of the body can be restored from the relevant reflex points on the feet.

This brings me to an important point which is that "it is the body that heals itself". The healer, practitioner, Reflexologist or Zone Therapist only facilitates this healing and unblocks the pathways for the body itself to do the work.

The body has the ability to not only heal itself through its electromagnetic field but it is also the world's most sophisticated pharmacy and capable of producing all kinds of drugs if the right conditions are present.

When blockages are removed, the body's pharmacy also gets to work. For example, it could be that the body has stopped producing enough anti-inflammatories to get your pain down. Zone Therapy can kick start the production again. Or the brain may have stopped or reduced production of endorphins which reduce pain or pain-related emotions. Zone Therapy can help.

How scientific is Zone Therapy?

Doctors will agree that the body has an electromagnetic field. This is proven by the fact that ECGs and EEGs exist and are relied on.

In this book, I am proposing that the feet have a direct effect on the body's electromagnetic field. I am of course saying that they have a positive effect and they are extremely accurate, in that certain zones of the feet correlated exactly to certain areas of the body.

For those of you who are even more skeptical than most and require concrete scientific proof, it would have been interesting if there was scientific studies that showed working on the feet has a direct effect on an ECG for example. That would have been very useful and a big step towards proving the theory of Zone Therapy and what Reflexologists believe in.

Guess what? There ARE scientific studies that show working on the feet have a direct effect on the electromagnetic field of the body as demonstrated by ECGs!

One such study showed that Reflexology had a moderate improvement on the heart's activity as measured by an ECG [7].

Another study has found that *"foot Reflexology may be used as an efficient adjunct to the therapeutic regimen to increase the vagal modulation and decrease blood pressure in both healthy people and Coronary Heart Disease patients"* [8].

In another study, volunteers participated in a physiological measurement of Reflexology on their feet. The tests were: EEG, ECG, continuous blood pressure, galvanic skin response (GSR), respiration from the nose and abdomen including nose respiration temperature, concentration of carbon

---

[7] Paul Joseph, U. Rajendra Acharya, Chua, Kok Poo, Johnny Chee, Lim Choo, S. S. Iyengar, Hock Wei, "Effect of reflexological stimulation on heart rate variability," Science Direct, 4 February 2004

[8] Altern Ther Health Med. 2011;17(4):8-14.

dioxide in nose respiration gas, blood flow and thermography. It was concluded that *"Reflexology showed good physiological effects"* [9].

Another study in 2003 concluded that: *"This implies that dynamics become less complex and the horizon of predicability increase during Reflexology"* [10].

And another: *"Remarkably improved ECG"* following Reflexology [11].

A study at the National University of Singapore on the effects of Reflexology on ECG found that: *"the dynamics of the heart become less complex during Reflexology"*. In other words subjects become more relaxed and potentially more receptive to healing [12].

These studies all show that there are scientific studies out there showing some effect on the electromagnetic field of the body as a result of working on the reflex zones of the feet. Science has shown that working on the feet does have a direct effect on the physiological functions of the body. Physiological functions are measured and correlate to electromagnetic activity. Electromagnetic activity can be accessed and positively interfered with from the feet.

The reflex zones used by reflexology are for the most part, identical to the reflex points used in Zone Therapy. By working on these reflex points, a Zone Therapist will be seeking to press harder and harder at each session. This pressing and "teasing out" of the tenderness means that as the session goes on and during subsequent sessions, the therapist is able to press harder at each session.

---

[9] "Physiological Measurements for Reflexology Foot Massage," Yoshio MACHI1, Chao LIU1 and Maki FUJITA21 Dept. of Electronic Engineering, Tokyo Denki University (Tokyo, JAPAN) 2Japan Reflexorogy Association Maki Fujita Reflexology School (Tokyo, JAPAN).

[10] Biyani A and P K SADASIVAN, "Nonlinear Analysis of ECG under reflexology stimulation", In World Congress on Medical Physics and Biomedical Engineering, 24-29 August 2003, Sydney, Australia, 2003.

[11] Zhongzheng, Li and Yuchun, Liu, "Clinical observation on Treatment of Coronary Heart Disease with Foot Reflexotherapy, 1998 China Reflexology Symposium Report, China Reflexology Association, Beijing, pp. 38 - 41

[12] http://www.eng.nus.edu.sg/EResnews/0406/rd/rd_5.html

If the problem is very bad, the therapist may only be able to put very little pressure on the reflex zone of the feet at first. After a few minutes, they can press slightly more. At the next session, they will start slow again but press harder a little later. The idea is that when the tenderness and feeling of granules on the reflex points are gone, the problem within the body will be gone. Once the Zone Therapy session is over, the body takes over and because some of the electromagnetic field of the body has been restored and repaired through zonal manipulation, the body will be able to heal itself a little bit more until the next session.

I mention therapist as I have not reached the point where you will be able to be your own therapist. For the purposes of this book, you will be working on your own feet if you are able to, so you will be the therapist. If you are very immobile due to your back pain and for example you cannot bend down or stretch, then a friend or relative will be working on you and he or she will be your therapist.

I speak a great deal about pain. The pain that the patient feels as a result of the therapist pressing the relevant reflex point of their feet is an indication of progress. If the patient feels no pain or discomfort, then real progress is not being made as fast as possible. My favourite patients are the ones with the highest pain thresholds! This way I can get on with doing my business, I will press as hard as they can tolerate and I know that their problem will disappear in record time. Zone Therapy on the feet with the probe being pressed as hard as the patient can tolerate, is the most effective method for getting rid of their back pain.

Don't worry if you don't have a probe either! I will be showing you what you can use which will do just as good a job as a probe similar to what I use.

Think of the discomfort on your feet from the probe during your session a little bit like training in the gym. If you are in the gym to build muscles, unless you push yourself very hard and do the heaviest weight possible, you will not build decent muscles fast. You will make some progress, better than not going to the gym but you won't get big and muscular.

The same principe applies to weight loss. If you don't push yourself out of your comfort zone in the gym, you won't see great results.

What you put in and the discomfort and pain you are willing to tolerate, dictate the results and the speed of those results.

Reflexologists often do not press very hard on the feet. They will help certain health problems eventually but no way near as fast as Zone Therapists. A Reflexologist with a strong set of fingers will give you much quicker results than one with weak fingers. This is a fact and something that people should consider when visiting a Reflexologist to help with a specific health problem.

In either case, I consider myself a very experienced Zone Therapist and my wooden probe leaves nothing to chance! If Reflexology with the slight pressure of the fingers has some activity or effect on the body, as proven scientifically, then can a bigger stimulation on the reflex points have a bigger effect on the electromagnetic and physiology of the body? I can tell you a definitive yes. Now let us find out what really is the main difference between Zone Therapy and Reflexology.

Zone Therapy's main differentiating factor to Reflexology is the use of a probe. In Zone Therapy, the practitioner uses a probe on the feet to eliminate problems in the body. In Reflexology, the practitioner uses their fingers on the various pressure points.

Due to the pressure of the probe and the way it can get into the problematic area, Zone Therapy is a far more effective method for alleviating problems than Reflexology. By this, I mean if you have a back problem and someone like myself puts the probe on your specific problematic spinal or back areas, you will see a great deal quicker results than a Reflexologist working on the same points with their fingers.

In addition, my Zonal Probing Technique puts pressure on very specific "rapid action" zones which produce even quicker results than Zone Therapy!

The other difference between Zone Therapy and Reflexology is that in Zone Therapy, a therapist like myself would only really work on your problematic areas and not the whole body i.e. not the whole of both feet. This was the Joseph Corvo method and one which I follow as I have seen the results first hand too many times and know that it is much more effective than Reflexology.

Having said that, Reflexology can be more effective in certain conditions due to the fact that the Reflexologist works not only on the problematic area but on the whole body. For example, if you have a skin disorder, a Zone Therapist may only work on your liver or a particular organ on the corresponding area of the feet. A Zone Therapist may concentrate on the liver only as he or she may think it is congested and needs re-earthing (zonal manipulation). A Reflexologist however will work on the whole body and therefore, so many other areas get worked on. Something that may well contribute to the healing process. Working on the adrenals, pituitary gland and kidneys etc may well help the healing process and further detox someone with a skin disorder.

Oh and just to confuse you a little bit more, many Reflexology and Zone Therapy charts sometimes differ in where they place some organs and body parts on the feet! But don't worry, fortunately for you, both disciplines agree on where the back and spinal areas on the feet are.

As far as back pain is concerned, nothing touches Zone Therapy in terms of speed of results, actual effectiveness and its non-invasive ways. I would never do Reflexology on someone with a back problem. In the early days, I would always go straight into Zone Therapy with my wooden probe. Now, I find Zonal Probing gives much quicker results. Throughout this book, I will be teaching you how to apply Zonal Probing for quick relief from back pain and in addition I will also show you other unique exercises, techniques and helpers.

Do remember that drugs and pain killers have side effects. Osteopathy and twisting of your spine can help you but it is often not permanent and can aggravate problems. Corticosteroid injections are most often a temporary relief. Massage on the back can give you more pain the next day. And of course surgery has its own risks and uncertainties especially when it comes to the spine, including paralysis. I am not saying don't try them. I am saying try them if you like and once they don't work, use the method in this book. Alternatively save yourself a great deal of time, pain, money and stress and just start Zone Therapy today!

Zone Therapy is unmatched in producing results and being safe. The problem is that not many people are trained in Zone Therapy! There are plenty of Reflexologists around but if you want to find a good Zone Therapist, then you are going to find that it's probably easier to find Big Foot or the Loch Ness Monster!

The reason for this is that there are no schools for training in Zone Therapy and the last Zone Therapist that I know of was the late Joseph Corvo, who was without doubt the master of Zone Therapy. Joe's passing means that there are no real expert Zone Therapists around that practice his unique methods.

A Google search for "Zone Therapist UK" will deliver all of... wait for it... zero results! A Google search for a Zone Therapist in the USA delivers only 1 major result which at first seems very promising with a Zone Therapist in most major states. However, the name Zone Therapist used is misleading as they are in effect Reflexologists and do not use a probe on the feet.

Not finding Zone Therapy to be popular does not detract from the principles and power of Zone Therapy. It is just one of those things. Ever since I met Joe and became trained in Zone Therapy, I always knew that what I did was very exclusive. In almost 25 years I have not come across anyone else that does what I do and knows the specific methods that I have learnt.

Personally, I do not have the time to practice on many people and this is why I have written this book for you. In the next chapter, I am going to explain to you just what is so different about my Zonal Probing Technique and why it is unique and not practiced by anyone else alive today.

5
The unique Zonal Probing Technique
and why it works

When I was studying the Legal Practice Course (LPC) at BPP Law School in the UK, we had around 10 students in each class. In the whole course there were maybe around 100 pupils. I would say out of them, there were probably 4 very clever students, not necessarily great lawyers, but extremely clever students. Then there were 1 or 2 that had a really good legal mind and you just knew they were going to be the super-star lawyers of the future.

When I was studying Reflexology, in a class of 20, there was one super-star student there. It was me of course! The rest were learning what they could and they would go on to become "qualified" and some would even open their own practice. Becoming qualified or going through the motions is very different from having natural talent and a "feel" for something.

I will admit that I was not and would probably never have been a great lawyer. I am very litigious and legal-minded and in my business career I am very successful at litigation but I would not consider myself a great lawyer. I am however one of the best Zone Therapists around today, if not the best. In 25 years, I have not failed to get some sort of positive response from the peoplel have worked on who have had back pain. And I am not talking about over a long period. I am saying that I have been able to produce positive results within 1 or 2 ten minute sessions.

What I am getting at is that you need to have a feel for something and be super-talented in your field. I am talented in law, business, music, documentary-making, photography etc but when it comes to Zone Therapy, my unique Zonal Probing Technique is quite simply unmatched. I am going to explain it to you. You will hopefully put it into action and then judge for yourself.

When it comes to back pain, I have been known to practice what I preach and will take on any challenging back problem and produce some noticeable relief within 10 minutes... on the spot!

Concentrate on the most problematic area

Perhaps the biggest problem with Reflexology is that it is just too "holistic" and tries to do everything. Ever heard the phrase "Jack of all trades and master of none?"

Reflexologists are trained in a specific way and they work on the whole body.

Traditional Reflexologists not only have way too much to do in their 30-45 minutes sessions, many of them are also not trained on specific problems.

It's a little bit like doctors. They are trained in everything medical apart from the one thing that is actually the cause of 99% of diseases: nutrition! On average, US medical students receive a mere 23.9 contact hours of nutrition instruction during medical school [13]!

Please don't get me wrong, I love Reflexology and have a great deal of respect for Reflexologists but when it comes to getting rid of certain problems, then Reflexology is not the one that gives very quick and noticeable results. This is especially so for what I call non-organs!

"What on earth is a non-organ?" I hear you ask. It is what is not classified as an organ :)

By this I mean the spine, back muscles and shoulders. Use my method for these non-organs and you will get incredible results that will astound you. Use Reflexology and you may not even see any results for weeks.

What I mean by concentrating on the most problematic area is if you have back pain, then concentrate on working on the back area of the feet and nowhere else.

Furthermore, when working on the back reflex zones of the feet, concentrate on the most tender, painful and problematic area.

---

[13] Am J Clin Nutr. 2006 Apr; 83(4): 941S–944S.

You need to be careful and not under-work it (as you won't see results) and not over-do it, as over-doing it may cause bruising and stop you from being able to work on the feet for a while. More on the exact method later.

So my first secret is that I always work on the most problematic area and I do not get distracted with other areas or what others believe are important areas to work on when it comes to back pain. Reflexologists will work on the whole spine. Zone Therapy tells you to work on a number of specific zones of the spine. The Zonal Probing Technique tells you to ONLY work on the most problematic and tender parts of the back and spine zones of the feet. They can usually be found by the patient; however this book will also give you these Rapid Relief Zones for specific back problems.

Reflexologists believe that other areas such as the adrenals and abdominal regions as well as back helpers are important and should also be worked on. This is not what Zonal Probing is about. You want results? You have come to the right place!

A few years ago I met with an old friend of mine for a drink in Gibraltar. He had just sold his company for £170 million pounds. At the time I was running my supplements company and also running a television channel which was costing me a fortune. The television company was taking a great deal of my attention and concentration and I guess in hindsight, I wasn't concentrating on my main business which was the supplements company.

My friend told me that one of the secrets of his success was that he would always concentrate on one thing at a time and the one that is the most important to him and most result producing - in his case, financially. His advice to me was to concentrate on the main "job at hand". I don't often listen to other people's advice unless they really know what they are talking about and you cannot argue with someone who is on the list of the richest people in the UK.

I eventually wound down the television channel and started concentrating more on my supplements company to great success. I don't necessarily think it was his advice as such but just something that made sense. Or maybe I did listen to him subconsciously!

I guess what I am getting at is that in many things in life, you will be a great deal more successful if you concentrate on one thing at a time and that one thing being the most important and relevant one to "you". When it comes to back pain, you must stick to working on the most problematic reflex points for the back. You must work on the Rapid Relief Reflex Zones. Listen to this consciously or subconsciously!

You need to tease the problem out

Let's say there is a man or a woman you are interested in. You ask them to dinner, they say no. What do you do next? If you are smart, you would approach again maybe with a smaller request. Coffee? A walk? A chewing gum?

Then maybe you get to go for a walk with them. Then you can push for a date and so on.

Life is push and pull. Yin and Yan. Effective Zonal Probing utilises this principle. Most of the time you cannot go hard and heavy and you cannot go too light... but you have to try and be persistent and focus on your goal. Not many worth-while things get achieved unless you have a goal and stay focused on it.

The unique method of Zonal Probing establishes a base and then pushes a little harder, then steps back, then pushes harder and carries on until the end goal: total elimination of back pain.

Reflexology does not use this "teasing" technique. No one does. I will do my utmost and will explain it to you very comprehensively in the next chapter but if I am to be honest, it is one of those things that needs to be experienced and felt first hand to get a real grasp of it.

My "teasing technique" differs from most Reflexologists in that I pay particular attention to the patient in so many ways and am always analysing how much more I can push or when I need to pull back. Reflexologists follow a script. I follow no script.

I take a history, analyse the client's speech, look for body language at all times, distract them at times with questions, put my hand on other areas of the feet for pain relief or further distraction. You don't need to know all these of course. You can just learn the Zonal Probing Technique in the next chapter and have very good success in getting rid of your own or a loved one's back pain.

Positivity pays dividends

I cannot begin to tell you how many times in my life positivity has paid off for me. I have achieved pretty much everything I always wanted whether financially, socially or emotionally by being extremely positive.

I am married to a wonderful, beautiful, intelligent lady because of my positivity.

I have a successful business career because of my positivity.

I have done impossible deals because of my positivity.

If you are positive in everything that you do, you will get there. I promise you.

The epicentre of the Parham Donyai Zonal Probing Technique is the positivity and absolute guarantee that your back pain will go away. I guarantee this as I have seen it too many times with too many people with all sorts of back problems. Your spine and your back muscles are like every other human. If the method works for them, it will work for you. Remember this and be positive. I am not asking you to take a huge leap of faith here. By introducing this unique Zone Therapy method I am not asking you to believe in aliens or martians. I am merely asking you to accept that your back area is reflected on your feet and that working on your reflex points can have a positive effect on the electromagnetic field of your body.

Once you start working on your feet, you will see for yourself that the exact problematic reflex points of your feet correspond to the same areas where you have your back pain.

If you have a back problem on your left side, you will see that the spinal areas of your right foot do not hurt when you press them. Only the left foot will hurt.

When you practice the method I will teach you in the next chapter and your back pain starts getting less and less after each session, you will start believing more in the method. Be positive and it will come. Nothing comes to negative people unless its just random. I repeat. **Nothing comes to negative people unless it is just random** and you don't want random. You want precise and self-generated.

The "two weeks per year" formula

As someone who has developed some of the best weight loss and muscle building formulas in the world, I am often asked questions like "how long will it take for this to make me lose 10 kgs?" or "how quickly can I put 5kgs of muscle on?".

The answer is: I have no idea! You see, I do not control other people's genes, discipline, goals, lifestyle, stress, social life, workouts and so on. How long, is very much dependant on them - but I do often give them an idea.

The unique Zonal Probing Technique can give you a very close estimate as to how long it will take for you to see at least a 50% reduction in your back pain. The formula is: **for each year that you have had your back pain, you need to have 2 sessions to see a 50% reduction in pain.**

You may say 50% is not so fantastic but I say it is. Imagine, your back pain which no one can cure or help you with gets reduced by 50% in just a couple of 10 minute sessions! You will be sending me chocolates, flowers and thank you cards for sure - my address at the end of this book and I don't eat chocolate :)

If you have had back pain for the last 6 years, I promise you that if you follow my method and the techniques described in the next chapter and that you stick to all the do's and don'ts in the following chapters, your back pain will be down by 50% in just 12 x 10 minute sessions. At the risk of over-promising, I can tell you from experience that it will be closer to the 100% relief mark. This is aimed at most people that have back pain, especially lower back pain but not those that have severe degeneration, physical abnormalities or major disease such as cancer.

If you have had back pain for 6 months, you will see between 50-100% reduction in pain in just 1 x 10 minute session of the "correct" method of Zonal Probing which I will shortly outline (come on Parham, get on with it!).

Manage expectations - Don't be impatient

My method is also about managing your expectations. I am a big believer in aiming big and never taking no for an answer but sometimes you have to be realistic.

Some people have such bad back pain that they may not be able to work on their feet the way I describe. Or maybe they live by themselves and have no one else to work on their feet. Or maybe their pain threshold is low.

My method and promises are based on all conditions being perfect and people adhering to what I say. Sometimes this is not possible. Also some people are different.

In my supplements business, we sell several Testosterone boosters. For some people, they kick in straight away and they get strong and muscular within a couple of weeks! For others, it takes a couple of months before real results kick in. This difference is due to many factors, many within the control of the person and many totally out of their control. Within their control are things like how they take the pills, how much alcohol they consume, how stressed they let themselves get (stress reduces Testosterone), how much they train etc. Outside of their control is their genes, their age, their own Testosterone blueprint, their own hormone production and so on.

Some people's bodies respond really well to Zone Therapy. I cannot tell you why and will not even begin to tell you that I know why! I don't! And there is no formula in determining who these people are going to be. If you are one of these lucky ones (and there are many) then I don't need to manage your expectations. You will have your first session and you will see and feel an incredible difference straight away.

My method is about constantly analysing and observing what is going on with regards to the feet themselves and on the spinal zonal areas of the feet. If a particular session or area gave very good results, then you will want to go back to that and do more work. Remember this and make a note of what worked well for you when you start your sessions. These are your Rapid Relief Reflex Zones.

If a particular session did not produce noticeable results but the tenderness in that relevant reflex zone is the worst of all the feet, then you need to go back to that area but re-adjust your expectations and bear in mind that you may be one of the ones that it takes a while longer to see results. Also it could be that you are afraid of a little discomfort and you were not pressing that area hard enough with your probe.

Do remember that if you have a long-standing chronic back problem, it is not going to go away over-night. You have to be realistic and you have to persist with the technique, just the way I persisted as a patient myself, even though I was experiencing a great deal of pain from Joseph Corvo's probe.

This same persistence is required from anything that will give you results over and above the norm. If you want to start running and you give up as soon as you start feeling out of breath, then you will never get fit.

If you want to build muscles and you just don't push heavier weights because it is painful or you stop going to the gym because results are not coming quickly enough, then you will never get muscular. If you want to lose weight but give up after a few 20 minute sessions on the treadmill, then you are destined to have excess weight and it is your own fault!

Zone Therapy is the same. Depending on how long you have had the problem, how you are applying the techniques in this book and how your own body reacts and heals, you may find that results appear in as little as one 10 minute session or it may take a few weeks.

If you have had a long term problem, be patient. Keep at it, stick to the techniques and results will come. Part of the uniqueness of my technique is the guarantee that I give you that you WILL see results and your back pain will be a thing of the past. Trust the method. Trust the probe!

It's in the probe!

Ultimately, the main facilitator in the abolishment of your back pain is the probe you will be using. It is the way the probe releases the electromagnetic blockages and re-earths your reflex points that are crucial to Zonal Probing working for you.

A Reflexologist will use their fingers in a continuously pushing or rotating method. Even a Reflexologist with very strong experienced fingers is not going to have the power and stiffness of a probe.

The probe has the ability to push and dissolve the problems that lie in your reflex zones, opening pathways for your own body's meridians to get into action and start the energy flow and healing process.

The helpers are part of the method that works

When I work with the R&D scientists at the LA Muscle laboratories in my supplements business, we always make sure that we use catalysts and delivery and uptake agents in all the supplements we develop. These catalysts make sure that the ingredients work faster and more efficiently, hence a more powerful and result-producing formula.

If you know what you are doing as a Zone Therapist, you will know what "catalyst" areas to work on and at what times and intervals, to make sure your method works speedily and efficiently. These catalyst areas are often referred to as "helpers". There are specific lower and upper back helpers that will speed up the whole process of healing and pain elimination.

Again, sticking to the first principle which is, always concentrate on the most problematic areas, sometimes these helpers are actually the primary areas that need to be worked on. How can you tell? You will be able to tell from the tenderness and reaction of the patient, which in your case will be you. If your lower back helper is more painful and tender than most of your spinal areas, then this is the area you will need to concentrate on and the chances are your back pain is going to go away quicker.

I have worked on many people with back pain and everyone is different. Their bodies, their postures, their beds, their abdominal support muscles and so on, are different. You cannot predict what happens. For the majority, the main spine areas will be the most problematic reflex points and need to be the primary areas to be worked on.

My method concentrates on working on these but at the same time concentrating on the helpers too, according to the results you will be getting. However you need to be open-minded and sometimes concentrate on the helpers first or pay more attention to them either at first or later on in your treatment.

Pay attention to the feet you are working on

Everyone's feet are different. Apart from people's pain thresholds, some people's feet are more meaty, some more skinny, some have veins, dry skin etc.

You have to be careful when working on your feet and pay attention to certain things. I will go over them in the next chapter but I just want to mention that my Zonal Probing method takes into account your own uniqueness and you must adjust accordingly. If you have a meaty foot, you will need to press harder with your probe. If you have varicose veins in a certain area, you may possibly need to work on the corresponding area of the other foot.

Now let's learn the 10 minute Zonal Probing Technique for curing your back pain...

6

How to perform the 10 minute Zonal Probing Technique on your feet

Human beings like to pigeon-hole things. It makes life easier.
"A simple life is a happy life". So they say!

When it comes to my unique Zonal Probing Technique for alleviating your back pain in just 10 minutes, I like to at least try and keep it as simple as possible. I know that as you get more into this nitty-gritty chapter, you may beg to differ but let's have a go anyway...

Reflexology and Zone Therapy Charts will vary in their complexity. Some will try and pinpoint the exact spot of each vertebrae on the corresponding area of your feet. This is really not necessary for Zone Therapy to work and if anything it makes it more complicated for you to work on your back pain.

Also, as far as holistic medicine and Zone Therapy are concerned, it doesn't really matter what your various scans, different diagnosis and doctors say is wrong with you and what area of your back has the problem. Zone Therapy will find the problem. Zone Therapy will do you no harm.

I don't want to sound indifferent but Zone Therapy could not be further from modern medicine. You are going to try it because modern medicine has failed you. Zone Therapy is not based on the same platform as modern medicine and has no correlation to it.

When I was writing this book, my agent asked me to get several doctors to endorse it - to give it more credibility. This didn't make sense to me! Here I am, telling you that Zone Therapy will fix problems that doctors with their years of studying and the extortionate fees often fail to fix. Why would they endorse Zone Therapy? And guess what? They don't! Personally I don't care and as long as you get well safely, rapidly and permanently, you shouldn't care either!

For our purposes, the 3 main areas to work on are: Upper back and neck, middle back and lower back. These are your general Rapid Relief Zones. We will be covering specific and highly effective ones with pin-point accuracy further down.

THE SPINE

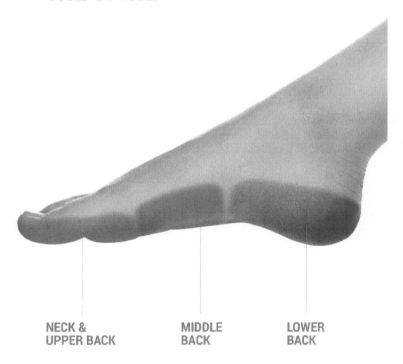

NECK &
UPPER BACK

MIDDLE
BACK

LOWER
BACK

The zones pretty self explanatory especially if you have very specific area-related back pain. Going back to my main principle of concentrating on the most problematic area, if you have lower back pain, then you want to be working on the lower back zone on your feet.

If you have back pain on the left side of your body, then you want to be working on your left foot. If you have pain on both sides of your body then you can work on both feet or either. Ideally, you should work on all the tender areas of both feet.

What if you don't know where exactly your back problem is? Or what if it is not just a specific region? That's simple! You have to work on the most tender reflex zone area of your feet which correspond to your back areas. This may be upper, middle, lower, some or all.

Start with the most tender area, always.

The other areas to consider are the upper back "muscles" and the lower back "helper". They are usually secondary areas to be worked on. However, if these are the most tender area of your foot and painful to touch or probe, then they should be your primary concern.

THE HELPERS

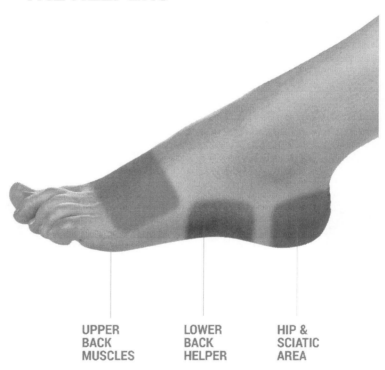

UPPER
BACK
MUSCLES

LOWER
BACK
HELPER

HIP &
SCIATIC
AREA

How to get hold of a probe

The probe is the most important instrument you can get your hands on for the purposes of this book. I have already explained to you that I made my probe from a wooden broom-stick, shaped and perfected it. You need not do this! You will need a probe, so let's show you how to get one.
Go to your local pharmacy or supermarket. Look for the section where they sell toothbrushes, toothpaste etc. Go down the aisle and get to the toothbrush section. Pick yourself an adult toothbrush, go to the counter and pay for it. You now have your probe!

The bottom part of 99% of toothbrushes acts as almost the perfect probe for alleviating your back pain using Zone Therapy. It would be better to have a shorter toothbrush with a thicker handle but this is really a minor point.

The end of your new toothbrush is your probe. You will be holding the toothbrush upside down, so you are holding the brush part with your hand (more like holding the middle) and you will be applying the bottom hard part of the toothbrush to the reflex zones of your feet.
Another alternative can also be a non-disposable razor such as a Gillette. The bottom part of most razors also act as a great probe. However, make sure you detach the actual razor part at the top before using it as you don't want to cut your hand.

Basic principle of Zone Therapy

Let's do a recap here. When the tenderness (or granule-like/girtty feeling under the skin) in the relevant reflex zones of your feet go away, your back pain in the relevant area of your body will go away. This is the case each and every time. Believe it and be persistent with the technique in this chapter. The more you persist and work on getting rid of the tenderness by applying the probe (toothbrush/razor end), the better your back will feel.

I know you are skeptical. It's natural to be skeptical as all this just sounds too good to be true. Don't take my word for it. Just try it for yourself. I promise you that after 1-2 sessions, you will feel a difference in your back pain. This will then be proof enough for you to carry on until you are totally free of back pain. Nothing worth-while comes easy. Remember that. You need to set your mind and persist. I have perfected and am delivering the no.1, natural, free treatment for your back pain which you can do in the comfort of your home. Give it a fair chance and don't be impatient.

If you had a choice and the luxury of a caring partner, then it is always preferable for your partner to learn the techniques in this book and apply them to you. But that's asking a lot of most partners!

Let's get started...

First session - Initial Phase of Zonal Probing

Have a good look around your feet. How do they look? Do you have a great deal of dry, scaly areas or are they generally in good health?

It is an interesting fact that in around 30% of people, where they have dry skin on a zone of their feet, it usually corresponds to a problematic area of their body. You may very well find that you have some dry areas or areas with thicker skin on your feet. They are actually a clue as to some of your health problems. They may well be around your heel (lower back) or side of your toe (neck).

Dry skin is only one sign. Discolouration, paleness or more often redness of the skin are also indications that the corresponding organ or body part may not be up to par - and even more interestingly, may be on their way to have a problem! Yes Zone Therapy can also tell you to a certain extent of upcoming ailments. But more on this in another book!

People with lower back problems can have dry heels. The heel area is very much related to the lower back and sciatic nerve. If you have dry areas here then you need to get rid of them before you can really get to work on your feet. Furthermore you cannot put a probe on the parts of your feet that have protruded varicose veins or broken skin.

I am not a chiropodist so cannot give you exact advice on how to get rid of dry skin, varicose veins or broken skin on your feet but you do need to address the issue before commencing your Zone Therapy sessions.

Soaking in a warm bath and using a strong file should help you with dry skin. Try and get rid of as much dry skin as you possibly can. The probe needs to have contact with your "live" skin and not dead dry skin. It cannot have contact with broken or injured skin and it cannot go over big protruding veins.

In your first session and your first time with your probe you may need to spend a little bit longer than 10 minutes to pin-point the right zones to work on and to get the hang of what exactly you are doing.

Look at the diagrams at the end of this book and the corresponding zones where you think your back pain is and start putting the probe on those areas. You have to press very gently at first as there may be a great deal of tenderness in some areas especially if you have had back pain for a long time.

Pay attention to the more boney areas of your feet as the tenderness may be much more in those areas. It is important to try and distinguish between the tenderness on your feet which is as a result of just putting a relatively sharp pointed instrument on the bone (the probe) and the deeper (and different) pain which is the result of problematic reflex zone areas. Do bear in mind that if you have had a chronic back condition for many years, then much of the arch of your inner feet may be tender to touch, reflecting much of your spine and back with problems.

Put the probe on an area and rotate it 3 times. Ideally, the rotation should always be clockwise. However in certain positions or with certain areas of the feet or for those who have mobility issues, clockwise may not be possible at all times. In such instances, anti-clockwise is OK. Move one or two millimetres up and do the same. In an ideal scenario, especially to be thorough in that first session, you need to start right from the bottom of your feet and heel and work your way all the way up. You need to do this on both feet.

After about 20 minutes, you will have a very good idea as to where the most tender and painful areas of your feet are. You only need to work on the back reflex zone areas which are along the inside curved part of your feet and the back muscles & back helper areas, as per the diagrams.

Once you have noted down the most tender areas of your feet, you need to start putting the probe on them in a more therapeutic way. Place the probe on a tender point of the foot, rotate it 10 times (ideally in a clockwise direction). Each time, it should take around 10 seconds. Don't put too much pressure, just enough so it is a little bit uncomfortable. Let go, move to the next area a few millimetres up or down, left or right and do the same. Rotate 10 times clockwise. Next area and do the same. Keep going up, down, left, right and coming back to the most tender zones of the feet.

Basically you need to cover the entire tender zones of your feet with the probe by going over them, again and again. I say feet, because for most people their back pain is on both sides of their body and so it is better to work on both feet. If your back pain is just on one side, then work on just that side - but it is rare for someone to have back pain solely on just one side.

My 3 minute warm up method followed by 7 therapeutic minutes - 3+7=10 minutes

You need to start gently and work on the various tender points with the probe for 3 minutes. This is a warm up and you won't be pressing very hard. You will be probing (pun intended!). After about 3 minutes of warming the foot up, you need to start pressing harder on the tender parts. In an ideal scenario you need to press hard enough just short of wanting to scream out loud. In other words, you need to press relatively hard on the tender reflex zones of the feet.

I have found this 3 minute warm up and 7 full on therapy minutes to be the most effective in getting rid of back pain. It is also the most effective with people who have a low pain threshold. Even if you were below average at math school, you will see that this adds to 10 minutes! This is your 10 minute back pain cure. You can just work on one foot even if your back pain is on both sides. I would however recommend to work on both feet i.e. 2 x 10 minutes, but that's up to you. 10 minutes will produce great results as it will kick-start your own body to start the healing process.

The business of you or your partner giving you a relatively high amount of pain and discomfort by working on these problematic reflex points of the feet is obviously not ideal. What can I tell you? It is a necessary part of the therapy. 10 minutes of relative discomfort a few times in your life vs a lifetime of degenerative, recurring, worsening back pain. You choose!

Don't be too put off if you have a low pain threshold or you just can't take 7 minutes of hard probing on your foot. You can press more lightly and give yourself less pain. The method will still work for you, though it may take a little longer to get rid of your back pain.

I am giving you the fastest and most effective method. That is the "press harder" and "feel more pain" method. If you can't take it, that's ok; go easier on yourself.

I guess because I have experienced the ultimate method personally myself when I had the back problems and in my practice days I have seen that those with higher pain thresholds get better faster, I am recommending this more hard-core method. But I understand that not everyone falls into this category and not everyone is as hard-core and impatient as me!

Once you have finished your first session, drink a glass of water. Always drink a glass of water after each session. You can get on with the rest of your day. It is obviously smart to heed the advice in later sections of this book as to what to do and not to do to help alleviate your back pain further and see it disappear faster.

Frequency of treatment

How often you should work on your feet is an interesting question. Most Reflexologists will see people once a week.

There are 3 reasons for this. One is time, the other is money. Most people don't have the money to see a therapist more than once a week and some don't have the time or both!

The other reason is that it usually takes a few days for the body to start reacting to the treatment. Remember, it is the body that does the healing and not the therapist. Zonal Probing only activates the body's healing mechanism and opens up the blocked meridians along the body's electromagnetic field. It is then up to your body to do the healing.

I would suggest that at the beginning, you stick to this once a week rule. You can monitor progress better this way too. By working on your feet once a week, you can see every week your back getting better and better and the pain getting less and less.

Sometimes, more is not better. In my supplements business, our scientists may include, say 300 mgs of L-Carnitine per day in a weight loss formula. Putting 900 mgs does not mean you will get triple the weight loss! The body doesn't work like that. You need to give the body the right triggers and then let it to do the work. Zonal Probing is the same. You need to work accurately and hard on the tender reflex zones of the feet and then leave your feet alone and let your body take over and to the healing.

For now, stick to once a week. Later on when you get more advanced and you know what you are doing, you can try working on the reflex zones once every 3-4 days.

I have been known to work on people such as those close to me or loved ones on a daily basis. Daily can be done but I suggest you stick to weekly at first and then once every 3-4 days for very chronic conditions.

Subsequent sessions after your first session

A week after your first session, you need to work on your feet again. The same 3+7=10 Principle applies here. You will start with a 3 minute probing as a warm up. You will press the various points to see where is the most tender. Chances are that it will be the same points as a week ago but you never know. The body has its own rules and its own ways of healing, so some of the areas may have moved or changed. In the 3 minute warm up you will find out where are the most tender parts and you will be teasing these areas by putting a little bit more pressure, then easing off, then a little bit more, then easing off and so on but not going in too hard.

After 3 minutes, start pressing the most tender areas with the probe, rotate 10 times clock-wise and then go to the next closest reflex point and so on. Start putting more pressure now and press it to a point where you can just about tolerate the pain and it feels uncomfortable. You don't want to have so much pain from the probe that it puts you off the next session but at the same time you need to take it to the point of the highest discomfort. This is the point where results are just around the corner.

You will be working on your feet like this for a few weeks. How long, depends on how long you have had the back problem for. The idea is to keep going in harder and harder at each session with the probe. You will find that you are having to press the probe harder at each session to get the same amount of pain and discomfort. If this is happening, then be happy as you are on the right track. I promise you that if this is what is happening, your back pain will be less and less after every session and a pain free back is getting closer.

You will reach a point where your back pain has totally disappeared. Depending on the individual you may find that all the tenderness has also gone from the problematic reflex zones of the feet. However for the majority of people, they will find that they still have some tenderness on their reflex points even if the back pain is totally gone.

From my experience, the majority of people will stop at this point as they don't see why they should carry on with relatively painful or uncomfortable Zonal Probing sessions when their back pain is fixed. However, if I was you, I would carry on just a little bit longer past this point. You want to make sure that your back pain does not return and whilst your back pain may have totally gone after a few sessions, if there is still a great deal of tenderness in the spinal reflex zones of the feet, then I suggest you carry on for a little bit longer.

When should you work on the back helper areas and back muscle zones?

A skilled Zone Therapist will go in and out of the various zones during a session. Let's say you have really bad lower back pain. I would primarily work on the most tender areas of the spine, generally on the lower inner curve of your foot, then lower down, along the side of you ankle and I would also go on your lower back helper area periodically. Remember, the inner curve of your foot is a direct reflection of the curvature of your spine and the 24 vertebrae.

The quickest results for you will always come from working the main Rapid Relief Reflex Zone areas on your feet, corresponding to where you have a problem usually on the spinal curve. As your weekly 10 minute sessions continue (for those who have a long-term chronic condition), you can start working on other areas such as the back **muscles** and the lower back **helper** areas, if they are very tender to touch. And do remember that I recommend 10 minutes on each foot for optimal results, so total 20 minutes.

This book is entitled the 10 Minute Back Pain Cure, because you will be able to cure your back pain in 10 minutes. However if you want better results and quicker results, then I would increase this to 10 minutes on each foot per session, especially if you are doing once a week sessions. You can also go up to 20 minutes on each foot per session if you feel there are too many tender areas and your back problem is spread out to too many reflex zones of your feet. Never do more than 40 minutes in total.

At the end of the day, there is no right or wrong here. NLP says *"Winning starts with beginning"* and I am a big believer in this. You would have already started to win and conquer your back pain by beginning and sticking to the methods in this book so whether you do 10 minutes every 3-4 days or 20 minutes every 7 days, you are still going to get amazing benefits and you will be on the road to healing your back pain.

What if you don't see any results at all, even after several weeks?

I have NEVER seen anyone not see any positive results from the techniques described in this book and I have been working on people since 1991. Admittedly when I started my various companies and became more successful I didn't need to work on anyone for financial purposes any more. However I have this urge to help people through Zonal Probing and have always worked on anyone who has had a health problem, especially back pain as it is so easy to treat. I can tell you with certainty that I have never come across this method not working for someone.

One of the worst cases of back pain I ever witnessed was a guy in my law class that had had surgery on his back. Even after surgery his back pain was so bad that he used to have to lay down at the back of the class, then he would get up and stand for a while, then sit and just move around constantly. The first time I worked on him I spent 5 minutes on his hands in the University canteen and he couldn't believe it. He didn't want to believe it!

I used to grab his feet during our lunch breaks and put my probe on them. His back pain gradually got better and better and he was a hopeless case as far as the doctors were concerned. The Zonal Probing Technique will work for you. Trust me, I am not a doctor!

You will see results, that is a certainty. If the results are not as fast and furious as you excepted, then there could be several reasons for this:

1. Your body just takes longer to heal.

2. You are not applying hard enough pressure with the probe (often the case). Or you may need to up each 10 x rotation to go up to 20 seconds i.e spend a bit longer on each zonal point so maybe rotate the probe 20 times.

3. You are not adhering to the other things in this book. i.e you are not protecting your back from further damage. For example if you are following the Zonal Probing Technique in this book but then going and deadlifting 100kgs in the gym or lifting heavy things incorrectly, then your back pain relief is going to go backwards or stay stagnant. During your healing phase, you have to stick to the rules which will be explained in the following chapters and give your body the chance to heal. This is a one time opportunity so stick to the rules.

7
Specific exercises to keep your back pain away

Whilst you are going to be doing Zone Therapy to alleviate your back pain, it is best to stay away from all exercise apart from the ones described below.

Exercise is generally good for you, however if you have a major back problem, or back pain, chances are that your back muscles are in spasm and contracting most of the time. Zonal Probing will be relaxing them but it is important to allow this relaxation to take place without additional pressure or contractions being introduced in the form of exercise.

Many exercises interfere with the positive effects of Zone Therapy. Running, football, weight lifting, yoga etc etc are all NOT RECOMMENDED when it comes to the period during which you will be performing Zone Therapy. Once your back is fixed and your back pain has gone and the spasms (which you probably don't feel as actual spasms) are gone, you can start doing the exercises of your choice again.

This advice does not mean that you stop moving. General movement such as walking is good for most back pain as it stops the back from seizing up and provides circulation and nutrition to your spine.

As you start doing Zonal Probing on your feet, you need to see how you go. This book makes a generalisation as I cannot be there for each and everyone of you. For example, if you are morbidly obese and you cannot even move much, then the below exercises may not be possible! You need to do the Zonal Probing Method and then perform the exercises as and when you are capable of doing them.

Sit-Ups

The basic exercise you need to be performing whilst doing Zonal Probing is a series of sit-ups, working towards building your abdominals, core and back muscles.

You need to wait until you have seen a slight positive shift in your back pain. This will usually come after your first or second session. When you have seen around a 20-30% reduction in your back pain, you need to start strengthening your core with sit-ups.

Lay down on the floor and put your legs under a low, heavy object such as your bed, so your feet are supported and kept down. Cross your arms across your chest and come up from the floor. You will probably need to bend your knees if you find this exercise difficult. Do as many as you can without experiencing too much back or abdominal pain. Once you feel pain, stop. Note down how many sit-ups you managed to perform before it became too painful.

Wait 3 days and repeat the same exercise again. This time, you will find that you will be able to perform more repetitions (reps). If you did, say 5 reps the first time, now you will be able to do 6 or 7 or maybe even more. Do as many as you can and then stop when it becomes painful.

Wait 3 more days and do more. The idea is to work your way to 30 reps with your arms across your chest. Once you have reached this point, you need to tweak the exercise slightly and start with your arms stretched out above your head and your legs stretched out on the floor. Now you need to come up with your arms (not on your chest). This is a more difficult version of the earlier exercise.

Do as many as you can up to the point of it becoming painful for your back or abs and then stop. Work your way up to 30 reps over the next few weeks/months.

If you are in a position to do 30 reps of this sit-up exercise, then your abs and core will be strong and you are on your way to support your back with your abs.

Push-up against the wall

You can start this exercise right now, every morning.

Stand against a wall, facing it. Place your arms with the palms facing the wall and rest your palms on the wall just above or in line with your head, arms apart shoulder width - like you are spreading for a police officer! Feet apart, shoulder width. Move your head and upper body towards the wall, as if you are doing a push-up against the wall. Lift up on your toes to take the pressure from your calves. Do as many as you can without it getting to be painful.

Once you have done as many reps as you can, turn around with your back facing the wall and stand about 0.5 metre away from the wall. Now you need to squat down almost to parallel, trying to push your buttocks against the wall without actually touching the wall, whilst trying to stretch your back as you are doing it. Do as many as you can without pain. Go down to parallel and then up again.

Count the reps on each and perform both exercises every morning and work your way up to more reps. Ideally you want to be doing 20-30 of each every morning but there is no rush to get to this level. Take your time and make sure you are building your way up to it without any pain.

On the push-up against the wall exercise you will want to be contracting your spine a little bit and on the squat against the wall you will want to be stretching the lower back.

Ab vacuum

Bend down with your hands on top of your knees - as if you are bending down looking at some ants on the floor!

Now pull your abs in as much and tightly as you can, hold for 5 seconds and then let go. Do as many reps as you can comfortably. This is a great exercise for not only making your abs stronger but also for your posture.

Perform the ab vacuum every morning and try and work your way up to 30 reps. It is important that this exercise is performed correctly with as much pulling in of the abs as you can manage. Over time you will be able to do more.

As with all exercises, it is important to perform them properly with a full range of motion and good form. It is better to do less with good form than to cheat and do more. You want to be building up your muscles and not just going through the motions. You want to "work" the muscle; slow movements, full contractions and full stretches.

Building your abs and your core are very important for the overall health of your back and spinal region. They will in time start taking 50% of the strain from your back.
However do remember that doing too much abdominal work, especially if it is painful can contribute to back pain, so take it easy if you get pain.

Back exercise to do when your back pain is gone

The above exercises can and should still be performed regularly to ensure your back and abdominal muscles are strong. Other exercises you can do are the following:

Hanging leg raises

Do hanging leg raises to strengthen your core and abdominal muscles. You need to build yourself up, so try doing as many as you can using good form without it becoming painful - even if it is just 1 rep! Wait 4-5 days and do this exercises again. Try and do a few more reps. Work your way to doing 20 reps.

You have to hang from something high up, ideally a machine in the gym specific for this exercise, and bring your legs up to your waist. At first you may need to have your knees bent but as you get better and stronger, you can have your legs stretched out.

Please bear in mind that if you get any pain in any exercise, you must stop immediately and not carry on.

Broomstick swings

Broomstick swings give you stronger serratus muscles, which are useful for having a strong core. You can do 2 sets of 10 reps every 3-4 days.

You have to stand straight, feet shoulder width apart. Put a broom-stick across your shoulders and turn to the left, then to the right and so on. Don't do it too fast and don't go too far to one side. Just turn enough so you feel the pressure on your abs and no pain in your back.

Crunches

Crunches and sit-ups can be performed in a variety of ways. You have been shown sit-ups above. You can add to your sit-up regime by doing crunches also - which are more or less the same as sit-ups. You can perform them in the gym or at home. You can find instructions on how to perform a variety of crunches on the Internet or from a personal trainer.

Deadlifts

Deadlifts are great for building your overall back muscles and for strengthening your back. Deadlifts are one of the core exercises used by powerlifters and bodybuilders.

You have to stand in front of a barbell with weight that you can comfortably handle for 8 reps, bend down, pick it up, slowly stand up straight with the barbell, hold the stood straight, extended position for about 3 seconds and then slowly lower the barbell down again.

You need to use a weight that is comfortable but not too comfortable and that you can do 8 reps, tiring slightly on the 7th and 8th reps. Then rest for 1-2 minutes and perform the exercise again.

The idea with Deadlifts and all major muscle building exercises is to try and increase the weight at each session to strength your muscles and build them to get stronger.

I understand that for most of you reading this book, you don't want to get big and look like a bodybuilder! That's fine, don't worry, you won't!
What I am trying to emphasise is that you do need to slightly increase the weights you are using each time you exercise to give your body reason to strengthen its own muscles.

The body builds muscles instinctively. If you lift something heavy repeatedly in the gym, the body tries to build a little bit more muscle as a protective measure to make sure it is ready against this heavy lifting. However, the weight needs to be slightly more than the previous session for this extra muscle building to occur.

If you start with deadlifting 5 kgs for example, you can work your way up to 10 kgs and then just stay at 10 kgs if you find that your back is getting too muscular for your liking - or if you find that your back is now strong enough. I can assure you that if you are Deadlifting 10 kgs, your back will not be too muscular but will be strong enough and closer to supporting itself and ensuring your back pain is kept at bay.

The Deadlift works a whole host of muscles and really is a great exercise. You will build your Trapezius, your Lats, your lower back and everything in between!

Many people have back pain, especially lower back pain because their backs are weak and their back muscles are weak. Weight training is a great saviour for many with back problems. Don't brush it off as just something for crazy meat-head male bodybuilders!

Exercises which are not so great for your back

Any exercise that puts pressure on your back by causing the vertebrae to contract on top of each other is not great for people who have a tendency for back pain. Number 1 on the list is running!

Having said the above, many people that I have treated have gone on to have normal lives which includes running.

I think you need to be cautious. Whilst you are doing Zone Therapy and getting well, you need to stay away from anything that makes your back pain worse or can be counter-productive. Running is one such thing.

When you are well and after a while, you can try going for a 5 minute run and see how you feel over the following 1-2 days. If all is well, you can start increasing your runs by 5 minute increments until you are running as long as you want.

8
Things to do and not to do to keep back pain away

I have been developing weight loss supplements along with a great team for close to 20 years now. In that time, we have developed some amazing products that genuinely help people burn fat and lose weight.

The supplements work well but how well they work really depends on the individual person taking them. If you give someone a fat-burning pill and they eat anything they want, don't do any exercise and don't take care of certain other things such as drinking water, then chances are that those pills will not do a good job.

For permanent weight loss, people need to change certain habits.

The same principle applies to my method of Zone Therapy and the promise to you that your back pain will be gone for good. You need to take care of certain things which directly affect your back pain. In this chapter, we are going to go over them. These are things to adhere to whilst you are doing Zonal Probing work on your feet to get the most out of your treatment. They are also logical and effective things to do to keep back pain away for the future.

Bending

If you have back problems, you should not be bending from your waist. You should not be bending down AT ALL. You should always try and bend from the knee. Bending down is very bad for your back and can really affect your progress.

If you have dropped something on the floor or you need to pick something up, bend from the knee.

Certain daily chores require bending from the waist. My advice is to try and not do them if you can. For example, making your bed requires bending from the waist. Try and get someone else to do it for a while or just don't make your bed! I know it sounds bad but if your back pain is really affecting your life, then little things really do affect progress.

Try not to bend down to brush your teeth. Protect your back. Try and keep it straight at all times.

Obesity

Your spine is supported by your back muscles and spinal erectors. The fact that back muscles support the spine is logical but only 50% of the equation.

In reality, your abdominal muscles are contributing at least 50% to making sure your spine is supported and that your body is balanced. Having strong abdominal muscles (abs) and no excess fat (big belly) is vital in alleviating back pain and keeping it away.

Don't get disheartened. If you are obese, you will still be able to get rid of your back pain using Zonal Probing. However, you need to know that as long as you are obese, the balance is not in your favour and a recurrence of back pain is always going to be a possibility.

Your back muscles need to be balanced out with your abdominal muscles to give them a rest and a break from supporting you.

Many people notice they start suffering from back pain as soon as they develop a bit of a belly and get a bit heavier in weight. Whether it is getting married (and letting go of yourself!) or starting a new sedentary job or whatever it is, if you find that you are gaining a belly, then chances are that you will be going towards the back pain route, if that has been a problem or is in your body's make-up. Add to that lack of exercise and the actual extra weight of carrying a belly and you can see why people who are obese or do not exercise can suffer from back pain, especially middle to low back pain.

This book has covered specific exercises to strengthen your abdominal and back muscles. You need to exercise!

I am very much aware that alleviating back pain through Zonal Probing is only part of the equation if you truly want back pain to stay away for the rest of your life. This is why several chapters of this book are devoted to other positive contributory factors and how to ensure they are tackled.

Keep your back warm

It is extremely important to keep your back warm. What we are trying to do with Zone Therapy is to open up the meridians and let energy flow through them efficiently and get your own body to heal your back. A big part of this is to get rid of back spasms and contractions. Your back needs to relax in order for healing to take place. Heat is always good for long term chronic back pain. Cold is bad.

If your back gets cold, this increases the spasms. Getting cold can happen from not wearing enough clothing, to catching a cold wind, going into a cold environment, not covering yourself in bed or letting something cold touch your back e.g leaning against a cold railing.

You need to keep your back warm as much as possible. This means covering up with a reasonable amount of clothing. Whether you are going out or most importantly in bed. Many people don't cover up well when sleeping. I would strongly suggest that whilst you have this back pain that you "totally" cover up your back area when sleeping. This means a long t-shirt tucked into pyjamas so there is no area that is exposed.

A cold shower is obviously a big no-no during the healing phase. Do make sure that if you can, you are bathing and showering daily with water as warm as you can take on your body. If you are bathing, make sure the bath is warm and stay there for a good 20 minutes. If the water gets colder, top it up with more warm water. You can massage your tender reflex zones of your feet with your fingers when you are in the bath. This will do wonders for you.

If you are taking a shower, make sure you get some warm water on your back for a good 10 minutes. It goes without saying that you must not get cold when coming out of the shower or bath as this will undo all the good the hot water has done!

Your bed and pillow are your best friends or big enemies of your back

No statement is truer when it comes to back pain than the above. I would even go as far as to say that a fair proportion of back pain is caused by your bed and/or pillow - usually the bed.

I understand that money is a limiting factor with the majority of people and so they cannot just go out and buy a new bed. However, if you are sleeping on a very soft bed, then you need to find an alternative if you can. Zonal Probing will still work and it will help with your back pain but you need to do something about your mattress if it too soft.

A soft mattress does not support the back properly and your back will constantly be in spasms and contracting. A soft mattress with light springs (you know, the type that you literally bounce every time you move) is very bad for your back and will be putting your progress back every time you lay on it.

On the other extreme, a very hard mattress is also not great as it can stiffen your back. The ideal is a mattress that is somewhere in the middle. I would advise "trying" a mattress for a few days if you can to see how it affects your back pain. One that makes you wake up with worse back pain in the morning is to be avoided at all costs. You will then just have to spend your 10 minute Zonal Probing trying to undo the damage caused by the previous night's sleep!

Pillows are also very important in contributing to or alleviating back pain, especially upper spine, upper muscular region of the back or neck pain.

Everyone is different when it comes to pillows. Some prefer soft and some hard. I would suggest you try a few different ones and see which one gives you the most comfort.

What you should take from this chapter is that your mattress and pillow are extremely important in your journey to back pain relief. You are quite literally spending 1/2 or 1/3 of your life on them so they must be supportive of your back in every way and not contribute to any spasms of your back muscles.

I cannot emphasise how important a good bed and pillow are. In some people, 80% of their problems are caused by a bad mattress. Think about that! Sleeping without a pillow is not good for the majority of people with back pain.

What is the ideal sleeping position?

As I have already mentioned, you have to bear in mind that with a book like this, I am generalising a great deal and writing for the majority of people with back problems. With this in mind, for most of the people who have back pain, sleeping on their abdominals (often referred to as "sleeping on your stomach") is bad for their back pain. This way of sleeping does not relax the back and further contracts the muscles, so in essence, sleep-time which is supposed to be relaxing and therapeutic is turned into a "tightening of the muscles" session.

This is applicable to the majority of people. If you are the exception and you find this way of sleeping helpful, then that's OK. I have known people to say sleeping on their stomachs actually helps keep their spine in check.

The best way to sleep when you have back pain is to sleep on your back or sleep on your side, in the foetal position. Many people find sleeping in the foetal position and pulling their legs in towards their abdominals very helpful.

This is trial and error but do pay attention and see what is the best for you. Stick to that method. If you find that sleeping on your abdominals destroys your back, then tape a tennis ball to your abdominals before getting in to bed and you will find that every time you end up on your front, the ball will hurt you and you will subconsciously turn around and change position.

Take your time getting out of bed. Don't rush up, get up slowly and make sure you do not put too much pressure on your spine when getting out of bed. Go slow.

Tight is bad, loose is good

My severe back pain was over 2 decades ago and it's difficult to truly recall and live the intensity of it. It was bad and it made my life hell at times, when I should have been having fun. If you are in the same position, I am sorry and hope this book can help you. At the time I didn't know that little things made a positive or negative contribution to my pain.

Tight things make a negative contribution to your back pain. Don't wear tight belts, tight trousers or tight skirts. Anything tight that presses against your back is not good. This includes leaning against uneven surfaces. Try and wear loose clothing and ditch the belt.

Massage may not be as good as you think

On the subject of direct contact with your back, as a whole, massage is not a good idea if you have a back problem. This has been my experience. Unless you personally (and as an exception) find a back massage helpful, I would suggest you stay away from it whilst you are doing Zonal Probing on your back. If nothing else, it will interfere with the process.

Although massage is considered as a relaxant, it can increase muscle contractions and spasms. Many people enjoy the "touching" aspect when they are having the massage but find that their back pain is much worse after having had a massage.

Later, when your back pain is gone, you can have as many massages as you like. Whilst you are performing the Zonal Probing Techniques of this book to overcome your back pain, you have to stay away from massages.

No other treatments whilst doing Zonal Probing

I think this is an obvious point but I will mention it anyway. Under NO CIRCUMSTANCES should you have ANY other non-medical treatment whilst you are doing Zone Therapy on your feet.

Obviously if you are under the supervision of a medical doctor or surgeon, you should carry on with everything they tell you. However, you must not have any other alternative or complementary therapy such as physiotherapy, osteopathy, chiropractic manipulation, massage, Reiki or anything else.

Firstly they will interfere with the Zonal Probing Technique described in this book and secondly they will skew your results and not show you clearly the progress you are making as a result of Zonal Probing.

CAUTION: When sitting behind a computer

Most of us spend at least a few hours a day behind a computer screen. Sitting and working behind a computer is one of the biggest reasons for low back pain in the developed world.

Your chair, it's structure, its height in relation to the desk, your posture, your stillness and how often you move are all contributory factors.

Ideally you should choose a chair that supports your spine. In other words, your spine is fully rested against the back of the chair. You should also choose a chair with some sort of support or foaming and adjustable mechanism for bringing it up and down. You should try and place your computer high enough so your posture is as perfect as possible and you are sitting up straight when working.

It is advisable to get up and move at least every 30 minutes. Stretch, walk around and make sure your back gets a break (not literally!).

Think of it this way, the more things you can do to take yourself back to the start of humanity (running, walking, exercising, hunting!) and the further away you are from sitting behind a computer desk, the better off you will be.

"Walking is man's best medicine" Hippocrates.

Pay attention to posture

Posture is extremely important when it comes to dealing with back problems. I can usually tell when someone suffers from back problems by just looking at them standing or walking.

People who have good posture generally suffer less back pain or at least their back pain is less severe. However, good posture is much like the chicken or egg scenario. Bad posture can lead to back pain and back pain can lead to bad posture.

Stand up erect, stick your chest out and make sure your back is straight. Do this when walking and when sitting. You need to make a conscious effort to do this until it becomes habitual. If you have had bad posture for a long time, you need to make a real effort here.

Obviously if you have a severe back problem, it may be difficult for you to correct your posture. Your muscles may be weak or hurting so take it easy and try and do it when you can, a little bit at a time and when you can remember. Do have it in mind to correct your posture eventually. Maybe try and set an alarm reminder on your phone every 20 minutes.

The World Health Organisation (WHO) puts a depressed mood as one of the main causes of back pain! I personally cannot see the correlation although I would say that those with a low mood often have bad postures. WHO also puts "age" as a leading cause of back pain. Obviously when it comes to age, there is not a great deal you can do! You can however reverse some of the damage done and unblock the blockages caused as a results of the years passing, through the use of Zone Therapy.

Small things add up to big things

There are a great deal of daily activities that can contribute positively or negatively to back pain. Here are a few to give you an idea and hopefully guide you to pay attention to similar things.

* Sneezing is terrible for your back if you don't keep your spine straight whilst you sneeze. If you sneeze with your back bent or to the side, it is like putting a ton of pressure on your spine.

* Don't wear high heels if you have a back problem. Not while we will be working on it.

* Don't slouch!

* Try and stretch but don't go past the point of pain. Pain is never a good sign and you should not push pain.

9
The 1 minute
back pain relief

There is a scene in the movie "There is Something About Mary" where the lead character played by Ben Stiller picks up a psychotic hitch-hiker who tells him about his great idea of how to make money.

The murderous psychotic hitch-hiker wants to do the 7 minute abs video to beat the very successful 8 minute abs video. Genius!

If 10 minutes are good for alleviating back pain, can the job be done in 9 or 8 or even 1? Actually no! However, what can be achieved in 1 minute is a very quick back pain relief - not a cure or total alleviation of back pain but a noticeable quick relief. In fact, this 1 minute technique used to be one of my party tricks and you can do it on yourself on others once you have learnt it.

Just to be clear, for the purposes of this book, you need to stick to the 10 Minute Zonal Probing Technique described previously. However if you are pushed for time or you want to just see some quick relief, you can apply one of several "quick results" methods below.

The Comb Method

The Comb Method can be applied as a 1 minute quick-action treatment or it can be incorporated into the longer 10 minute technique too. It is effective either way.

For this method you need to get yourself down to the pharmacy again! This time, walk down the brushes & comb aisle and pick a strong comb. You want to be using the big teeth of the comb for this. You can also try a metal or horse comb, which you can buy from the Amazon website.

Place the big teeth of the comb on the tender reflex zones of your feet which correspond to your problematic back areas. Rotate 5 times clockwise. Move on to the next area a few millimetres on either side.

The comb is a very quick and effective way of relieving back pain. The comb method works amazingly well in less than 1 minute to alleviate back pain especially if you are pressing on the exact zones. The smaller, sharper numerous teeth of the comb can get into areas that the probe may miss or may take longer to get to.

The comb method will never replace Zonal Probing with the probe in totally alleviating back pain because you can never press too hard with the comb; not enough to really go deep and permanently remove the blockages on the reflex zones. You won't be able to as the comb will dig into your foot and break/damage the skin!

You have to be careful with the comb and press just hard enough to "feel it" on your feet but no more.

The Chinese Burn!

Another party trick of mine is the Chinese Burn. Grab your wrist with the thumb and middle finger of your other hand. Hold it tight and rotate the wrist left and right i.e. giving yourself a Chinese Burn with the circle created by the thumb and middle finger of your other hand.

This Chinese Burn works directly on the Sciatic nerve and lower back regions and gives amazingly quick relief from lower back and sciatic pain. If your back pain is on the left, then grab the left wrist. If on the right side of your body, then grab your right wrist. If both sides, then do one wrist at a time. Spend a minute, holding the wrist tight and rotating left and right, in 10 second increments.

The Chinese Burn is also very effective for period pain and women's menstrual pain!

Access your back and spine areas from the hand reflex points

I have purposefully neglected telling you about the reflex zones on the hands as I didn't want to confuse you too much. The fact is that your hands also have the same reflex points that correspond to your spine and back areas. It is more difficult to access specific points from your hands as they are more compressed together and the results are not as long lasting. This is why it is always better to work on the feet.

However, you can get pretty good back pain relief by working on your hands in under 1 minute.

Place the thumb of your right hand on the bottom part of your thumb area of the left hand and work your way up making very tiny steps with your right thumb. Make sure you keep pressure on the hand with your thumb at all times. Work up and then use your thumb to work your way down. Then do the other hand. Your spine is along the side of your thumb/thumb base. The top of your thumb near your nail (on the side) is your neck and the base of your thumb near your wrist is your lower back.

By now, you should be an expert so you will know your particular problematic area, as the reflex zones corresponding to it on your hand will be tender and painful to touch.

Other body parts that can contribute to alleviating back pain

As I have already mentioned to you, I have tried to keep the methods in this book simple and tried to stick to the strongest method as the primary fixer for your back pain - this being the probe on your feet.

In this 1 minute back pain relief section I have given you some extra relatively strong techniques to quickly get rid of back pain when you are on the go or when you are pushed for time.

I don't want to confuse you but I don't want to short-change you either so I am going to tell you about 2 more techniques that can greatly contribute to the alleviation of your back pain.

The tongue

Your tongue has many reflex points on it, corresponding to your various body parts. For a quick 1 minute "alleviating workout" on your spine, stick your tongue out and press your upper teeth on the lowest parts of your tongue. Keep them there for 10 seconds and then move a little bit higher and lower, pressing for 10 seconds again.

You will instinctively know where to put more pressure and keep pressed for longer as they will be your tongue reflex points corresponding to your back and spinal areas and will be a little tender. Though you won't feel pain as the tongue is nothing like the feet in terms of pain.

The ears

The ears also have reflex points (or acupuncture points) corresponding to your back. The curvature of your spine is inside your ear along the curvature of your ear.

I think by now you know that you should be working on your right ear if your back pain is solely on the right and vice versa. You should also know that this is rarely the case and most back problems are central or on both sides to some extent.

You need to grab your ears, pinching closest to where the back/spine acupuncture points are and give them a good massage for 1 minute. This is a great way for relieving back pain, though not as effective as foot and hand Zone Therapy.

10
How nutrition can help with back pain

"Let food be your medicine and medicine be your food". Hippocrates

It's probably a bit of a stretch for you to think that your diet and nutrition could be affecting your back pain! Right?

There is a connection between your diet and your back pain and I will explain how and what you can do to ensure your back pain is further relieved by eating the right foods and avoiding the wrong ones.

Eating the wrong foods can cause "inflammation" in your body and eating the right foods can reduce this inflammation.

Inflammation is your body's immune system response to problems within the body such as injury or infection. The inflammatory process involves a hugely complex biological series of molecular and cellular signals that alter your physiological responses, resulting in symptoms such as pain and swelling. Your body is constantly trying to deal with a whole array of things and certain organs such as the adrenals are working hard to bring down inflammation.

Long term chronic inflammation is caused by persistent activation of your inflammatory molecules. Food can be the cause of this.

Foods that are bad for you

It has been found that diets which contain trans-fats and saturated fats are pro-inflammation [14].

If your diet consists of fried foods, foods with animal fat, junk foods, chips, crisps, pastry, chocolate and foods which contain high saturated fats, then chances are you are not helping your back pain.

---

[14] Basu A, Devaraj S, Jialal I: Dietary factors that promote or retard inflammation. Arterioscler Thromb Vasc Biol 2006; 26(5): 995-1001.

Excess carbohydrates have been found to also be pro-inflammation [15].

Most people consume large amounts of carbohydrates such as pasta, rice, white bread and potatoes without thinking much about their effects on the body. Not only can these carbohydrates contribute to obesity, they can also increase inflammation in the body i.e. they can be directly contributing to your back pain.

More and more scientists are coming around to naming sugar as the new enemy of the body. Humans were just not built to consume as much sugar as we do these days. Too much sugar gets the body to send out cytokines, immunity messengers, which communicate cell to cell, usually as a response to some immune system problem such as inflammation.

The fact that too much sugar releases cytokines is a clear signal that too much sugar can be causing or increasing inflammation i.e. not helping your back pain.

Sugar should be avoided or at least reduced. This includes actual sugar and hidden sugar in foods. Sugar-ladened soft drinks are also an obvious no on the list; whether it is sugary sodas or sugary drinks. Their substitutes are not much better as they usually contain artificial sweeteners such as Aspartame which have also been associated with inflammation (and a whole host of other diseases!).

Alcohol is another big no-no when it comes to inflammation. Not only does alcohol turn to sugar but it also has a tendency to leak through the intestinal tract, causing inflammation in the body. Back pain is only one of the problems alcohol contributes to. Alcohol is also well-known to cause liver problems as well contribute to other auto-immune system diseases such as Psoriasis.

---

[15] Esposito K, Nappo F, Marfella R, et al.: Inflammatory cytokine concentrations are acutely increased by hyperglycemia in humans: role of oxidative stress. Circulation 2002; 106(16): 2067-72

Milk should be avoided or reduced, at least for the period of Zone Therapy treatment. Milk is not something that agrees with most people and many people are intolerant of the lactose in milk. Milk, especially semi or full fat milk can cause inflammation and act as a barrier to healing your back pain in as quick a time as possible.

Celiacs are intolerant of gluten as it causes huge inflammation problems for them. If you are a celiac, then gluten is obviously one to avoid. However even if you are not a celiac, gluten can be an inflammatory food and often is.

If you can, I would strongly urge you to avoid foods with gluten whilst you are doing Zone Therapy. Again for the sake of clarity, the Zone Therapy methods in this book for alleviating your back pain will work regardless of whether you avoid gluten or milk. The advice in this chapter is to speed up your healing.

Gluten-free pasta and bread are everywhere these days, so it is not difficult to get hold of them.

MSG (found mostly in fast foods) and caffeine are also known pro-inflammation ingredients so should be avoided or reduced.

Foods that are good for you

The so-called "Mediterranean Diet" is anti-inflammation and highly recommended to bring down inflammation in the body [16].

Higher intakes of the omega-3 fatty acids such as Alpha-linolenic acid (ALA), Eicosapentaenoic Acid (EPA) and Docosahexaenoic acid (DHA)) are associated with decreased inflammation (through their biomarkers) [17].

[16] Babio N, Bullo M, Salas-Salvado J: Mediterranean diet and metabolic syndrome: the evidence. Public Health Nutr 2009; 12(9A): 1607-17.
Giugliano D, Esposito K: Mediterranean diet and metabolic diseases. Curr Opin Lipidol 2008; 19(1): 63-8.

[17] Giugliano D, Ceriello A, Esposito K: The effects of diet on inflammation: emphasis on the metabolic syndrome. J Am Coll Cardiol 2006; 48(4): 677-85

The number one constituent of the Mediterranean Diet is olive oil, high in polyunsaturated fats which are known for being anti-inflammatory.

Fruits and vegetables are another obvious choice when it comes to eating healthier and reducing the body's inflammation. They also contribute to making your blood more alkaline which is good for health.

Most nuts are generally good for inflammatory problems as they are high in essential fatty acids which are anti-inflammatory - not if you have a nut allergy though! Peanuts in particular contain Arginine, which is an amino acid shown to be highly anti-inflammatory [18].

Seeds such as sesame and sunflower are also great anti-inflammatories.

Many B-Vitamins are great anti-inflammatories. If you were to consume more vitamin-B-rich foods you could be helping your back pain. Vitamin B6 in particular has been shown to be a great anti-inflammatory food [19].

B-Vitamins can be found in poultry, pork, fish, eggs, vegetables, whole cereals and bread.

Vitamin C is also a great-anti-inflammatory [20]. Vitamin C can be found in oranges, dark peppers, broccoli, strawberries, mango, pineapple and papaya.

Foods that are known for being anti-inflammatories are carrots, beets, sweet potatoes, cherries, berries, grapes, pomegranate, watermelon, cinnamon, ginger, rosemary, garlic, the active part of turmeric known as curcumin or turmeric itself, onions, oregano.

---

[18] Salas-Salvado J, Casas-Agustench P, Murphy MM, Lopez-Uriarte P, Bullo M: The effect of nuts on inflammation. Asia Pac J Clin Nutr 2008; 17 Suppl 1: 333-6.
US Department of Agriculture, Agricultural Research Service. USDA National Nutrient Database for Standard Reference, Release 22. 2009.

[19] Friso S, Jacques PF, Wilson PW, Rosenberg IH, Selhub J: Low circulating vitamin B(6) is associated with elevation of the inflammation marker C-reactive protein independently of plasma homocysteine levels. Circulation 2001; 103(23): 2788-91.

[20] Seaman DR: The diet-induced proinflammatory state: a cause of chronic pain and other degenerative diseases? J Manipulative Physiol Ther 2002; 25(3): 168-79.
Jialal I, Singh U: Is vitamin C an antiinflammatory agent? Am J Clin Nutr 2006; 83(3): 525-6.

11
Weight loss for a stronger back

Over the years I have had a fair bit of experience in the area of weight loss. I first began developing weight loss supplements with a top team of scientists in 1997. Some of the formulas we developed went on to sell in the millions and help many people keep their weight under control.

I know that the subject of weight loss supplements is another area where people are skeptical so I don't particularly want to concentrate on that. I just want to let you know that I have read a great deal of scientific papers on weight loss and I am very aware of ingredients and foods that contribute to weight loss.

What I also have is a great deal of experience in diets and exercises that work well for weight loss. My sports nutrition company has sponsored some of the top athletes in the world and many of these athletes and bodybuilders need to lose a great deal of weight fast. For example, when a bodybuilder is going to compete on stage, they usually lose a huge amount of weight in just a couple of months.

Weight loss needs to be healthy weight loss, so I am not suggesting that you follow a bodybuilder's diet, though it would give you astonishing weight loss!

In 2009, I started The Active Channel, which rapidly became Europe's number 1 health & fitness channel. This was a full-on television channel on the European SKY network and was costing me almost £100,000 a month to run! We moved the channel online and on 24/7 Apps a few years later.

What the Active Channel gave me is even more experience in working with some of the world's best athletes and sports-persons. We have had some of the world's top sports stars and even some well-known celebrities on the channel. Many of them shared their weight loss success stories with us.

Let's move on to what this chapter is about. In order to alleviate your back pain and have a strong, healthy back, you need to have a strong, healthy set of abdominal muscles and a strong core.

I am not suggesting for you to have a six pack - not unless you want one! What I am suggesting is to ensure that you have a strong set of abdominal muscles that support your back and your spinal erector muscles. I am also suggesting that if you are obese or slightly overweight, you need to lose the excess weight which could be putting additional pressure on your back.

You are what you eat - of course!

We are all lazy! It's as simple as that. We are getting lazier and lazier. We are doing less and less exercise and eating more and becoming generally unhealthy.

Every morning you have a choice as to start the day eating the right way, being healthy and losing weight, yet you choose the croissant or the coffee with caramel and cream or the donut and generally just the wrong sort of foods.

If you start the day by giving your body the wrong signals, your body will carry on in the direction of those signals. Image a train that comes to a junction. Left is the junk yard and right is the beautiful forrest. If you take the left track in the morning, you are going to end up the in junkyard! You cannot suddenly turn back!

What you put in your mouth will have a direct effect on your health and your weight and potentially, your back pain! You may be lucky or you may be young and you may not see the effects right away but boy, wait until you are a bit older or you get a health problem! Then you will see that the foods you eat really affect your body.

Unfortunately doctors are not really trained in nutrition so they don't tell you this, however so many diseases are caused by what you eat; almost all in fact.

As for being obese and over-weight, it is caused by what you eat and your lack of movement and exercise.

Diet v Exercise

The equation for weight loss is simple. It is the opposite of the equation for weight gain!

When you eat more than what you use up, you put on weight. To lose weight you need to do 2 things. Firstly you need to start eating less generally as well as eating more of the right foods and less of the wrong foods. Secondly you need to exercise and move more to get rid of the weight you have accumulated.

However, before all this, you need to work on your mind. If you do not know why you want to lose weight and you are not motivated enough, your weight loss will be temporary and will not last. This is the sole reason why so many diets fail as they are usually a temporary measure in the mind of the dieter. In fact, just using the word "diet" alone is recipe for failure! A diet gives the impression that it is short term and you can go back to you old ways. You need to think of it as a new way of life and a new permanent healthy regime.

When you start eating healthier and exercising, you will start losing weight. I have to bring my experience into this at this point as I am all too aware that progress is often slow or comes to a sudden halt so keeping motivation high is very important.

As with anything, if human beings (especially this day and age) don't see results rapidly, they lose focus and lose faith and get close to giving up. Any weight loss regime that will eventually help with your back pain needs to give you relatively quick results, yet be safe and long term. A big ask!

Weight loss supplements are an obvious catalyst you can use but I will save selling them to you for another time :)

You need to follow a healthy, basic, earth-like diet that works well and you need to start increasing your activity levels.

What to eat

This is the million dollar question! The answer actually lies in your past or rather humanity's past. Whilst it is true that people are living longer, it is also true that people used to be leaner, more toned and more defined many years ago. The Paleo or the Cave-man diet is popular these days! It takes us back to how we used to eat. Many diets are popular these days in fact, so it's hard to choose! Atkins, Dukan, South Beach, Mountain Shack and so on.... ok, I made up the Mountain Shack one but you get the picture.

Let's start with why you want to lose the weight. You want to lose the weight because you want to look great, feel great and be rid of your back pain for ever. You want to start a whole new regime and a whole new you and live your life the way you were meant to live it and by looking good and not being in pain all the time.

Put a few photos of your old thinner self on several walls in your house or put photos of someone you like, admire or aspire to look/be like. Get some motivation going.

Everything starts with the mind. If you have it in your mind, you will achieve it but you need to be focused and you need to be persistent.

The general diet for losing weight is one where you start reducing all the foods that you were not meant to eat. Also you will be reducing portions too. In addition, you will stop all the grazing during the day that most of us seem to do these days. It's actually quite easy to do and once you get in the routine, you will see that not only do you see results, but you also start feeling better about yourself.

Your only hold-back right now is your mind, so you need to get your mind-set right and when you feel you are ready, let's start living the life you were destined to.

Mornings and breakfast

The mornings really depend on you. I know that most diets or healthy eating manuals recommend having breakfast to set you for the day and so on. I think this is very much dependant on the person. If you are generally not hungry in the mornings and you are fine going the morning without much, I don't see why you need to add calories to the equation. If you can have something that fills you up and you are OK, then do it.

However, this "filler" cannot be high GI carbohydrates such as pastry or sugars! Choose from one of the following for breakfast:

* Tea or coffee with no sugar or sweeteners

* Skimmed milk

* Low fat cheese

* Eggs

* Lean ham or salmon

* Porridge with skimmed milk - if you are very hungry

Mid morning can be some form of protein such as an egg, low fat cheese or a latte with skimmed milk. You can also have a handful of nuts such as almonds which curb appetite. The trick is to eat a little bit of protein "before" you get hungry. Once you get hungry, it may be a bit late to control your appetite.

Never go shopping on an empty stomach!

Lunch and dinner

I am going to put lunch and dinner together to simplify things for you. You can choose from the following for lunch and dinner and mix it up for variety.

* Lean meats, steak, tuna, chicken, turkey, fish, tofu, eggs

* Salads

* Vegetables

For example your lunch can be Tuna and salad. Or steak and broccoli. Dinner can be chicken and salad and so on.

I have removed carbohydrates (carbs) from lunch and dinner as you will see much better results in weight loss if you could just avoid carbs. This IS possible for most people if they follow a high protein diet and eat protein "before" hunger strikes.

Once you get hungry, it is much more difficult to avoid carbs, especially simple carbs like pastry, sugars and fruits. You know the feeling: you are hungry and you start grabbing every sweet thing in sight!

If you were to choose porridge for breakfast for example, this is usually enough carbs to see you through the day especially if you are having protein and vegetables (which have carbs in them).

If you usually get hungry mid afternoon or late at night, you can have some nuts or low fat cheese, eggs, low fat lean meats such as lean ham or a no-fat protein shake with no sugar.

By the way, fruits are generally OK and good for you but if you want quicker results in weight loss, I suggest avoiding them or reducing them for a few weeks. You will still be getting your fibre and vitamin and minerals from vegetables.

The other key weight loss accelerator is water! I know you have heard it a thousand times before and you probably ignore it but drinking water is KEY to losing weight. Water is the ingredient that shifts the fat out of your body. Drinking water is essential to the movement of fatty deposits out of your system. By water, I mean clean fresh water and not fruit juices or tea/coffee.

This is not a weight loss book and I don't want to spend pages and pages on weight loss. The aim of this book is to alleviate your back pain and as I have mentioned, losing weight, being lean and building your core and abdominal muscles can be extremely helpful in stabilising your back muscles.

When you follow the above healthy eating guide, you will start to rapidly lose weight. If you have a medical condition or suspect one, then it is advisable to seek your doctor's approval before starting any sort of new eating regime especially one which reduces your so called "normal" carbohydrate intake.

When you have reached your ideal weight, you can start adding more carbs to your diet but you need to keep their levels lower than before. You can also have protein only days to further reduce/maintain your weight. This is where you eat nothing but protein for one day a week. So breakfast would be no/low-fat cheese, lunch could be a steak and dinner would be a tuna steak or chicken breast.

Things to avoid when trying to lose weight are:

* Fruit juices, sodas, sugary drinks, drinks with artificial sweeteners

* Fried foods, anything with saturated fats

* Junk foods, fast foods, pizzas, chips

* Pastry, sweets, croissants, donuts

* Eating late in the day and too close to sleeping

The best exercise to lose weight

This is another area which I consider my speciality! I have worked with so many fitness athletes and bodybuilders over the years to get them lean and in shape for competitions and events. This has given me a unique insight into what works and what doesn't.

Weight loss is easy. The key and the real secret lies in your mind-set. Like most things that are difficult to stick to, exercising for weight loss needs you to take a step back and see why you want to lose the weight. You then need to find the strongest reason and blow it up in your mind and keep it at the front of your mind at all times. Visual imagery and physical imagery around the house and your place of work will help.

To lose weight, you need to 1) start doing cardiovascular exercise in 2) your Target Heart Range (THR) and for 3) long enough. These three go hand in hand and are the 3 secrets to losing weight through exercising.

The best cardiovascular exercises are:
* Fast/brisk walking
* Running/jogging
* Cycling outdoors or stationary cycling
* Rowing
* Stepping (The stepper in the gym)
* Cross trainer (gym equipment)

Dancing, weight training and moving around the house are not ideal for weight loss as they don't stick to rule number 2, which is keeping you in your Target Heart Range (THR).

Your THR is where you optimally burn fat and your body starts accessing fat stores for energy rather than using up foods you have eaten or even worse, using up your muscles for fuel.

The more muscles you have, the more fat you will burn whilst resting - so the last thing you want is to lose muscle mass!

To simplify, your THR is where you are exercising and not totally out of breath and not too comfortable. In your THR if someone asks you a question, you can answer them but you will be panting and pausing every few words.

The third ingredient to a successful weight loss exercise regime is for you to do it long enough and stay in your THR long enough. Most people do 20 minutes and then they stop or switch to a different exercise. You don't really burn fat in the first 20 minutes of exercising!

The ideal scenario is to stay on the one machine or stick to the one exercise and try and do it for at least 45 minutes in your THR.

Depending on how much weight you need to lose and what your state of health is, it would be good to work your way to 60 minutes of cardiovascular exercise in your Target Heart Range, 4-5 times a week.

As to what is the best time, mornings on an empty stomach is a good time but don't worry too much. As long as you do it and stick to the regime, any time is good.

12
The 10 commandments
A recap!

In this small chapter, we will do a recap of what you need to do cure your back pain.

1. Set your mind first

Firstly, you should be proud of yourself. You have decided that living with back pain is not for you and you want to do something about it. You have already shown that you can set you mind to change your life!

Now set your mind to put what you have learnt in this book to practice. Believe that you will rid yourself of your back pain using the techniques in this book and commit to doing at least the 10 minute Zonal Probing sessions.

2. Avoid things which make your back pain worse

Top of the list is bending down, lifting heavy, getting cold and so on. Avoid anything that hurts your back either consciously or habitually over time.

3. Start Zonal Probing on your feet with a probe as soon as possible

Whether you choose a tooth-brush end or shaving razor end, you can start working with the probe on your feet as soon as possible.

4. Pay attention to your nutrition

Start avoiding inflammatory foods and try and eat more of the foods that help bring down inflammation

5. Start doing sit-ups

Once you have done 1-2 sessions on your feet and your back pain is around 20-30% less, start doing sit-ups to strengthen your back and your abdominal muscles.

6. Do a 1 minute back pain relief exercise when you can

Perform one or all of the 1 minute back pain relief exercises when you can, when you are pushed for time and when you are out and about. They will really help you and will further reduce your back pain. It is good to try and get rid of pain any time possible so you start getting used to a life without pain.

7. Build up your core and abdominals

Once you are better, start doing the specific exercises in this book for building your back and core.

8. Exercise

Once your back pain is 100% better, start a regular exercise regime.

9. Reduce your weight

If you have excess weight or are obese, start the weight loss regime to get rid of the weight.

10. Don't forget and be grateful

Humans have a great tendency to forget. I am urging you not to forget! Once your back pain is gone, do not forget how it went away and don't get complaisant. Don't start bending the wrong way, lifting incorrectly, showing off in the gym, gaining weight, not exercising, eating badly and so on.

If your back pain comes back a little bit, do the 1 minute back pain relieving exercises.

If you do something wrong and you hurt your back, start Zonal Probing on your feet with your probe immediately. The sooner you start, the quicker you will get rid of the pain.

There you have it. I am proud of you. I really am. You have managed to do something that 50% of people fail to do and that is to follow something through to the end. You have managed to read this book to the end and I am sure you will succeed in alleviating your back pain. If you have reached this far, you are a winner and you will go on to apply the techniques in this book and alleviate your back pain.

I really hope Zone Therapy and this book's unique Zonal Probing Technique will be a turning point in your back pain and in your life the way it was for me. As far as back pain is concerned, Zonal Probing is "the one" you have been searching for. Congratulations, you found it!

Specific Problems and their related Rapid Relief Reflex Zones

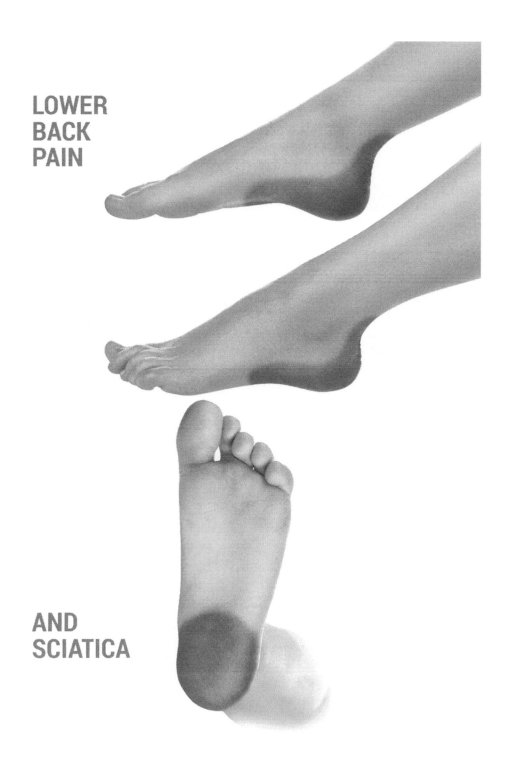

LOWER
BACK
PAIN

AND
SCIATICA

MIDDLE
BACK &
MUSCLES

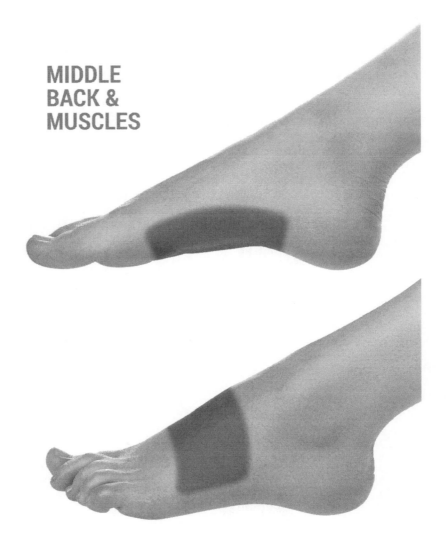

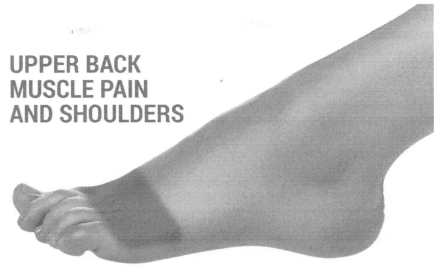

UPPER BACK
MUSCLE PAIN
AND SHOULDERS

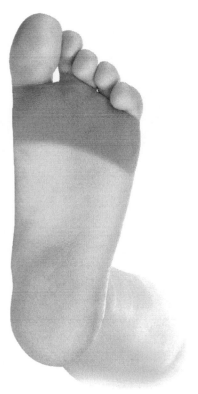

NECK PAIN

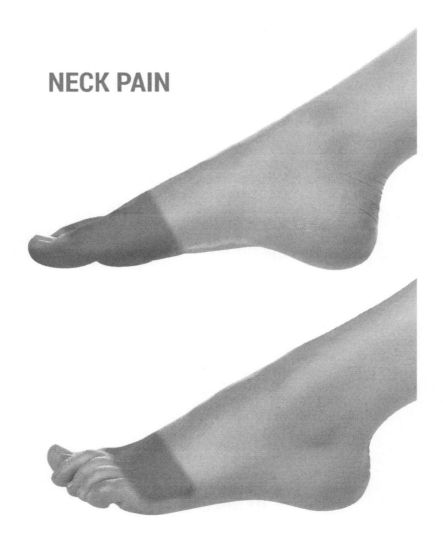

Glossary

3+7=10 Minutes
3 minutes of warm up Zonal Probing, followed by 7 minutes of firm, direct Zonal Probing.

Helpers
Other areas of the feet with zones which can influence problematic areas in the body. They are not directly connected to the area in the body but have a strong influence on healing.

Meridians
Meridians are energy channels in the body. They are pathways along which vital energy flows.

Neurolinguistic Programming (NLP)
A unique method for achieving success, altering your beliefs and achieving your goals.

Probe
An instrument that helps you to accurately and firmly work on different Reflex Zones of the feet. The end of a toothbrush or the end of a non-disposable razor can act as a suitable probe.

Rapid Relief Reflex Zones (Rapid Relief Zones)
Specific and direct areas of the feet that correspond exactly with where your back pain comes from. They are the most tender points in your Reflex Zones.

Reflexology
The ancient practice of working on pressure points of the feet and hands to relax the body and alleviate health issues.

Reflex Zones
Areas of the feet corresponding to areas of the body.

Target Heart Range (THR)
Your optimum fat burning range. It is when you are panting during exercise. THR for weight loss is 60-70% of your max Heart Rate. 220 minus your age give your max Heart Rate.

Two weeks per year formula
Where it will take 2 weeks' worth of Zonal Probing to get rid of back pain for each year you have had it.

Zonal Probing
The unique method described in this book of applying a probe, rotating it 10x clockwise on the tender Reflex Zones of the feet.

Zone Therapy
The system of applying a probe to specific Rapid Relief Zones of the feet.

For more information, please visit: zonetherapy.co.uk

Printed in Great Britain
by Amazon.co.uk, Ltd.,
Marston Gate.